T0121848

EXPOSED!
THE WEIGHT LOSS INDUSTRY
WANTS YOU TO BE FAT

*Primitive Health and Fitness expert
reveals his 9 secrets to quickly and
dramatically transform your body*

DAVID BEARES

authorHOUSE®

AuthorHouse™
1663 Liberty Drive
Bloomington, IN 47403
www.authorhouse.com
Phone: 1-800-839-8640

© 2013 DAVID BEARES. All rights reserved.

No part of this book may be reproduced, stored
in a retrieval system, or transmitted by any means
without the written permission of the author.

Published by AuthorHouse 2/11/2013

ISBN: 978-1-4817-1417-4 (sc)
ISBN: 978-1-4817-1882-0 (e)

Any people depicted in stock imagery provided
by Thinkstock are models, and such images are
being used for illustrative purposes only.
Certain stock imagery © Thinkstock.

This book is printed on acid-free paper.

Because of the dynamic nature of the Internet, any web
addresses or links contained in this book may have changed
since publication and may no longer be valid. The views
expressed in this work are solely those of the author and do
not necessarily reflect the views of the publisher, and the
publisher hereby disclaims any responsibility for them.

CONTENTS

PILLAR TWO

TRAINING

PILLAR THREE

TREATMENT

My Story

OW IN THE WORLD DID I become the Primitive Health and Fitness Expert? Well, from a very early time in my life there were two big factors that made me who I am. One, I was always intensely connected with nature. I had an obsession and connection with Native American culture and spirituality. Two, I was someone who always questioned pop-culture beliefs.

I was a fairly smart kid, but I can't say that I've ever enjoyed school very much. I found it boring and constricting. I would much rather have been outside playing with my friends. It's still funny to me that I worked through a master's degree because the classroom experience has never been that pleasant to me.

It was my passion for the earth, traditional wisdom, and my desire to question norms that led me to think outside the box. I was born with a strong skepticism for "new is better."

The big transformation happened in my mind and life

about 15 years ago. I had two very painful experiences one summer, one being the loss of my last, and closest grandparent, who we called Daddy Don. (I swear he wasn't mafia.)

Raw and in a ton of emotional pain, I took off for Monhegan Island in Maine to hang out with my best friend Tim who was working for the summer in a restaurant on the island. There wasn't a lot to do there, but Tim gave me a book to read, <u>Ishmael</u> by Daniel Quinn. I took that book and devoured it on the cliffs looking over the Atlantic.

As I read, something opened and shifted in me. All of the loose thoughts and feelings I'd had from my childhood had something to root onto. I had context for my thoughts about the earth, our place and responsibility as humans in this lifetime, and the way to heal as people. But I didn't have a vocation at this point. I had nothing to apply this new passion towards.

Over the next five years, I spent time living adventures. Almost two years working in the mountains of northern Georgia at a wilderness camp for incarcerated youth did a lot to strip me of my youthful arrogance. I believe every 20 year old needs to do something that challenges the oversized ego of their teens. This was mine.

My time in those mountains was powerful, and although I felt outmatched by many of these kids with extremely challenging needs and life circumstances, there were a few amazing times where my impact on their lives was apparent. This time in Georgia was really what helped me grow up fast, and it also gave me the strength for the next stage of my life.

I went on a life altering adventure. Something that tested my tenacity, that whipped me physically and mentally. Something that showed me what's on the other end of hard work. A reward that can only be gained through sticking with something physically grueling and making it to the other side.

This adventure was a 2,160-mile hike of the entire Appalachian trail from April 2nd to September 30th of 2001. Nothing in my life, besides watching my son Max being born, has impacted me and opened my heart like this hike.

After the first month of the hike, when at least 70% of the people had quit, I saw something different in the eyes of those who stuck with it. There was a glimmer of passion and an understanding that you could only get if you stuck with it. Those who stopped short of the full hike will never what they missed.

As I was cruising along, hiking swiftly through the woods of Vermont I had an overwhelming thought, a clear insight into my steps beyond the trail. Without explanation, I knew that I was ready to find a vocation, some sort of work where I could apply my love of health, the earth, and traditional wisdom to a career.

It was a very weird image, because it felt like a knowing, like I was seeing a picture of myself in this new career. But I still didn't know what it would be.

Less than a month after finishing the trail, I found the direction for my passion and skills at a school right near my family home. The September after the hike I started acupuncture and headed down the path of bringing primitive health and wellness tools to the community.

I was, yet again, learning another ancient system in the form of traditional medicine. This integrated the cycles of nature that I'd experience during my time in the woods with the health systems of the body in acupuncture. It all led me to being the primitive health and fitness expert and roots everything I do today.

Over the next 10 years, this passion morphed into the business and wellness system I've built: **39 Minute Workout**. The thoughts, tools, and system in this book are the culmination of all the information I've put together from a wide variety of sources and experiences.

This is the same system of treatment, training, and nutrition that my family lives by, and the same system I've taught to hundreds of local residents in my Columbia, MD practice. This book is my chance to finally share this with a wider range of people.

What I really hope for you, the reader is nothing short of a personal transformation. I will seek to rip apart the lies that the modern food, health and weight loss industry have sold you for decades now. I will seek to bring you back to a simpler, time-honored wisdom that puts you back in control of your health and wellness.

If you choose to follow what I'm teaching, I believe you'll be equipped to transform your health and that of your family.

INTRODUCTION:
WHAT'S WITH PRIMITIVE?

I 'VE CHOSEN TO USE THE word primitive here for several reasons. I'm aware that the word "Primitive" is offensive in the paleontology world, so I need to make it clear. I have COMPLETE RESPECT for primitive/traditional/indigenous cultures.

In fact, in many ways I consider them far more advanced than we are today. For one, they knew how to live in a way that was supportive of health. They ate what they were supposed to, used their bodies as designed, and often had deeper sense of culture and family than we do in our modern, fractured society.

Primitive is the term I chose because it speaks to Simplicity, not backwardness. Primitive ways are inherently simple and beautiful. They're not junked up with dogma. Primitive ways of living were based off survival, so they lived on the earth dictated by the laws of nature. Today, we eat to stuff ourselves or to satisfy our taste buds. Primitive people nourished themselves.

We have a skewed sense of the struggle primitive cultures lived under. Of course it really comes down to which tribe, which region, and which time of history. But that view of "life as struggle" is a bit out of whack. I would say that it was life in balance. It was biology and environment in balance. Again, if you'd like to read a story of where things went wrong, I would start with Ishmael!

WHO AM I WRITING THIS BOOK FOR?

You'll see in most of the stories and details, I'm writing to women. Partly, I did this because 75% of my clients are women and I know their struggles and strengths very well.

But really, the information in this book is appropriate for anyone; man or woman, young or old. I'm writing what I consider to be timeless and ageless information. There is no age, sex or race that would be exempt from the Primitive Health and Fitness movement.

In fact, my intention is to show that these are the rules of Treatment, Training and Nutrition that were followed by most of our ancestors in some form. It is my belief that in this crazy world of stress, terrible food and inactive lifestyles, we HAVE to get back to our Primitive ways fast if we want to remain a viable society.

LAYOUT OF THE BOOK:
TREATMENT, TRAINING AND NUTRITION

Y OU'VE SEEN ME REFERENCE THIS twice now. These are what I call the Three Pillars of Health. I have structured the book around the three pillars. With each, I have started by ripping modern/conventional wisdom apart. First I tear down the false beliefs of nutrition, and then follow by showing what I believe to be the simple and Primitive truths of nourishment.

I've done the same thing in Training. I've shown two disturbing patterns in modern exercise that are keeping people from living healthy lives. I've then laid out a framework for appropriate exercise, again, based on our Primitive needs.

In Treatment, I've simply made a case for traditional ways of treatment. I've shown why you should choose to replace modern healthcare with traditional forms of medicine. To make traditional medicine your primary care, and to save most modern medicine (short of physicals and regular check-ups) for "emergency care," only to be used when deeper pathology (such as cancer or a broken bone) arise.

I've ended with a bonus chapter where I present what I call the Health Portfolio. This is a way to reframe your mindset around health. I will encourage you to stop seeing money spent on health as an expense, and to start viewing it as an investment. You don't call stocks, bonds and investment property a burdensome expense. Yet, when people spend money on exceptional health, they often see it as a burden. It's time we reframe this whole conversation.

It's time to launch in. READY???

CHAPTER #1

EXPOSED!!!
WHY THE WEIGHT
LOSS INDUSTRY WANTS
YOU TO BE FAT

I WANT SO BADLY TO HELP people in this culture get well. When I'm out in public and I see how many people are heavy, sick or visibly unhappy, it makes me sad. Actually, when I see it with children, it makes me irate. Obesity has become a health epidemic, and carrying excess body fat has become the norm.

The situation is even direr when you look at children. The activity level and nutrition for children in our culture should be a crime. It is treated as perfectly acceptable for a parent to say, "My kid only eats chicken fingers and pasta," as if that's the way children are and have always been. Really? So at the turn of the 19ᵗʰ century, are you telling me that children had their own meals made for them every night, devoid of nutrients, monochromatic (that's one color), and wrapped around sugar and other carbs?

No way was this the case. Children might have been fed slightly different foods then adults up until now, but they weren't fed the junkiest, health destroying, useless food their parents could find. And parents surely didn't go making extra meals for them to be "happy" because they just won't eat the broccoli and rice you made.

We are setting ourselves up for an epidemic even more severe in the coming decades as these kids with no base of athletic skill, who only eat only sugary white food, begin to raise their own children. And hey, we raised them. It's our fault. And the proof comes in a very concerning statistic that you, too, have probably heard all over the news: **Adults currently have a higher life expectancy than their children for the first time in history.**

So it is time that we STOP this insanity, get back to our athletic roots, get lean and healthy, and start eating real food again.

My mission is to help people get back to the simple truth that is accessible and within us all. It is also to take us back to time-honored truths around nourishment and movement, not the latest scientific study telling us that soy is great and meat is the enemy.

When I look at the weight loss industry, I see the opposite of my mission. People are being sold nutrient devoid food, quick fixes, and even worse, dangerous solutions like diet pills and stomach staples.

I'm talking about Big Industry, made up of food, pharmaceutical, manufacturers and media who's primary mission is to make money, not to support our health. They are all part of the multi-billion dollar per year industry selling you fat loss products that offer nothing to improve our situation as a culture.

It pisses me off because I don't trust their intentions, and nor should you. Without going into a political discussion, which I'm not looking to do here, I want to make a simple point.

The weight loss industry needs you to be fat. They need you to buy their quick-fix toys, pills and videos.

That's exactly what I am **EXPOSING** here. I don't believe that these industries have your best interests in mind. I believe that their focus is to Sell Stuff.

They have driven the trend that's made us a chronically overweight culture, and they aren't doing a lot to help us get out of it either. And call me cynical, but I don't believe they actually want you to get better. If they did, there would be much fewer and better solutions on the market for you to use.

If the fat loss industry really wanted you to have the best solutions possible, it would have certain qualities. The products:

» Would be simple and easy to follow

» Would be reproducible (work for the masses and

have long-lasting success, not just flash in the pan success)

» Would help us get slimmer as a society

» Would support the best to rise to the top and sell for decades, because real solutions aren't trends. They are truths that hold up to time.

EXPOSED!

What the industry ACTUALLY teaches YOU:

» **Indulge-– here's food that tastes good, who cares if it's bad for you**

» **Make it quick-– stop cooking, stop spending time with family, just get it done– this trend led to decades of people who a) don't know how to cook b) don't eat <u>real</u> food c) have major health problems**

» **Eat food that's not food (dye, genetically modified "food", etc)-– it's yummy**

» **Don't believe those environmental nuts, science lab food is fine for you**

» **When something goes wrong with your health... voila, here's your quick-fix**

In a matter of a few decades, the industry has taken away one of the most basic components of being human, our ability to feed ourselves. I grew up in the 80's and 90's, and what was the big movement at that time? Save time, make everything easy.

Well, they did just that. And now we have a generation of people who don't eat real (unprocessed) food, don't know how to cook, have no connection with where their food came from, and then don't understand why they have cancer and heart disease.

EXPOSED!

We love to blame people who are "lazy and suck off the system" in this country. But when you look at what we've been taught-- don't take responsibility for your health; just cover it up with quick medical fixes; don't take time to cook and eat with your family; save time and stay busy-- you see that the industry has actually taught us over decades to be lazy and irresponsible. It makes for good consumers, people who rely on what the industry is selling.

This has impacted us on so many levels. The obvious one is our health and weight, but it's also our connection with family. We've all been told over and over that food is something that should be rushed, and it should taste good (no matter what the quality or where the TASTE is coming from). So now our family units suffer, because we've spent decades not spending time at the dinner table sharing good food and conversation. But yeah, we're saving time.

The industry that I blame most for the horrible pattern of obesity is the Food Industry. To me, they are the worst offender. The food industry's ONLY goal should be to provide the best food for humans that is both 1) beneficial to the people consuming it and 2) beneficial to the planet. PERIOD!

The food industry has almost nothing to do with providing good quality. When I do grocery store tours with my clients, I teach them about preservatives, dyes, fillers, additives, and so on. And I always ask the same question when I show them these over-processed, adulterated products; "Who is this food good for?" Not you!" This is good for production and shelf life, PERIOD. The stuff that's being put in our food has **NOTHING** to do with making you healthy.

Notice that they don't call it farming anymore. They call it Agri-Business. An important factor that I believe you should be worried about.

Pink Slime is a perfect example of the Agri-business and their lack of concern for the consumer. Jamie Oliver brought this disgusting product to light on his show, **Food Revolution**. This is basically the nastiest and dirtiest parts left over from cattle, rinsed in ammonium hydroxide to make it "safe and palatable."

Miraculously, after pink slime was exposed in national media coverage, McDonalds grew a conscience and banned it from their beef. Hooray! I guess I might ask why this was ok in the first place. But I'm just some crazy health advocate.

For you the consumer, this points out a very important fact. You need to care about where you eat and what you eat if your goal is to be healthy. And I want to make it ABSOLUTELY clear; I have no issue with meat. I just believe it should be fed and raised in a way that would make it suitable for consumption.

So again, if your goal is to be lean, healthy and to have a great quality of life then start that process by being an informed and proactive consumer.

Let's Raise Money to Find a CURE

I'm walking a tight rope with this one, and I really don't want to upset people. So let me make it clear what I'm poking at. If you've lost a loved one to a disease, or God forbid have a child who suffers from a disease/disorder, I completely understand wanting to raise money for a cure. My business, **39 Minute Workout**, supports a local charity, the Ulman Cancer Fund, because we believe in their cause and have worked to raise money for them.

BUT, I have a bone to pick with this concept of constantly wanting to find a cure for every disease. A cure for Type-I diabetes, great, let's do it. A cure for Type-II diabetes? We have one. Control what you eat and use your body the way you're supposed to. We don't need a "cure" for preventable diseases; we need prevention and lifestyle changes.

And every time I hear about another fund raiser for heart disease, I think to myself, if we would spend all this money on getting people to eat real food again, protecting our environment, and promoting preventative medicine, we would save so many more hundreds of thousands of people than we would by raising more money for poor multi-billion dollar pharmaceutical companies to "find a cure" for every disease known to man.

On top of raising money for cures, you've also got insurance companies footing the bill for gastric bypass, but doing nothing significant to help the patients make real lifestyle changes. So again, most just gain the weight right back. Again, there's something wrong when gastric bypass if covered by insurance when prevention is the real "CURE" we need.

We don't need a cure for every disease out there, especially when most diseases we suffer from are caused by poor lifestyle. Most of my clients I see in the acupuncture room or our training classes are suffering from pathology caused by poor eating, sleep, stress, and lack of exercise. Everything I've put in this book from my Three Pillars of Health (Treatment, Training, and Nutrition– more on this later on) would be more suited for attacking the diseases we suffer from than constantly dumping money into searching for cures.

We Don't Get Off Scot-Free Either

Our human vulnerability affects us as a consumer and has played a role in this trend too. We, as a society, don't get off scot-free. We've bought everything they've sold us. We've bought the useless tapes, the next goofy tool, toy or machine that doesn't work, we have taken the pills, gotten the surgery, eaten the unhealthy food, chosen to stop eating at the dinner table with our family, and trusted food from a box instead of whole foods.

That's exactly what they are preying on. The weight loss industry knows that we want a quick solution. Sure we desperately want to reach our goal– lose 20 lbs, get off all our medications, etc. – but there's a little secret we may not want to admit. WE DON'T WANT TO WORK HARD TO GET THERE.

I see this every week in my practice. I do consults with clients who have big goals that mean so much for their lifelong physical and mental health. Many are truly willing to put in the time and effort. They just don't know how to do it on their own. But there are always a few people who don't even want to meet their support team halfway. These people want the goal, but they don't want to do anything to get there.

So before you look to blame the fat loss industry, are you willing to do your part to make the necessary changes in your own life? Are you fired up and ready to take back your health? If so, that leads me to my next question…

Will You Help Me Drive the Next Major Health Trend?

I want to drive the next major health trend. Will you join me by committing to following these principles?

This is my BIG life goal. To make this happen, I will need you to join me. Some would say the problem is too big, but that is never a good reason to be wimpy. What's at stake is our health and happiness. I say let's take back our health.

I've written the Primitive Health and Fitness Revolution Manifesto to describe the role you have in making this change a possibility.

Here's is the Primitive Health and Fitness Revolution Manifesto:

» **I will accept personal responsibility**– As a consumer, I accept the fact that I am solely responsible for what I feed myself and my family. While there are many temptations and pitfalls along the way, I am ultimately responsible for my choices.

» **I will be a wise consumer**– I will demand better products from the farmer to the grocery store. I will know where my food comes from, and I will seek the best possible foods and sources that my budget will allow.

» **I will educate myself on the Primitive Rules of nutrition and exercise**– I will commit to getting the movement and nutrition that my body needs. I will step out of my comfort zone and explore the exercise that my body needs, even if it seems foreign to me at first.

» **I will be a role model for my family and others around me**– We cannot make a Primitive Revolution unless we make it viral. We have to spread the word, educate our friends and family, and be a great example.

I want to help **Revolutionize** the way you live. I want to give you the simplest roadmap to absolute health; one that is rooted in tradition and nature.

So here we go!

PILLAR ONE:

NUTRITION

CHAPTER #2

WHY MOST OF WHAT YOU'VE LEARNED ABOUT NUTRITION IS WRONG

NOTICE THE WORD I USED here: Nutrition! I didn't say Diet.

It seems that whenever we are talking about eating or weight loss, the Big "D" word comes out. Let me make it clear, **Diet** and **Nutrition** have very little to do with each other.

A diet denotes deprivation-- running a calorie deficit so that one can lose weight. Nutrition is about nourishment-- getting everything your body needs to be healthy and perform well.

I truly believe the Fat Loss industry has us focus on diets and not nourishment for the exact reason I **EXPOSED** them in chapter one. Their number one focus is not helping you get lean and healthy, it's selling products. And the diet crazes that follow one after the other are a major factor in the perpetual wheel of fat loss and diet products.

If Nourishment Were the Focus

If the focus were on **nourishment**, the world would be a different place. If media covered nourishment and not fad diets; if stores sold **Nourishment Plans** (like the one I'll describe later in the book); if pharmaceuticals focused on nourishing supplements and not wonder drugs, we wouldn't have an obesity epidemic.

It would be virtually impossible for fast food restaurants to exist. It would be almost impossible for weight loss pills, goofy workouts and dull food-in-a-box eating solutions if we were educated on **nourishment** and not diets.

I will say this several times in this book. You need to completely shift your focus if you want to be lean and healthy. And pardon me for my harsh wording, but I'm trying to make a point here.

Do not approach weight loss like a "fat person trying to lose weight." You should match your eating and lifestyle to the way a truly healthy, lean person lives...or as I'll describe later...the way your primitive ancestors did. Approach weight loss like you are aligning your habits with someone that has already reached the goal you'd like to achieve.

I believe this simple shift in thought can be a powerful

tool in re-shaping your purpose and goal here. I cover the mindset shift that has to happen in Chapter 8.

Most <u>Experts</u> Are in Too Deep

I've met some great dietitians and nutritionists, but just like the weight loss industry, so much of what comes from the "expert" is impractical and not rooted in history.

What I mean here is that their advice is hard to follow. It's often based on very recent science, yet lacking in historical perspective. It's often wrapped around dogmas (inflexible systems of diets and weight loss) that make it painful or dull for the client to follow like strict calorie counting systems.

I find that in many industries, experts have gotten in so deep that they lack perspective. They have spent too much time looking at the science of this moment or the diet of this moment.

Consequently, the advice of many of the experts is, in my mind, awful and impossible to follow. I'll get into a discussion about why I don't believe in calorie counting, and why I think you should NEVER lose weight this way.

But it's also the types of food they promote, like soy as a miracle food, and the fact that they tend to follow short-term trends in nutrition science and not time honored truths about humans and food. So if you follow the advice of many pop-culture nutritionists, you will get tossed around in a flurry of whatever miracle food or diet is the answer today. The fad of the week!

This trend tends to confuse the heck out of the public.

How many times do you hear someone say, "I have no idea what I'm supposed to and not supposed to eat. It seems to change every day."

100,000 Years

NO! The human body's needs do NOT change every day. Science changes every day. The next scientific study or power food highlighted in your favorite magazine changes every day. (Is it acai or pomegranate I should eat now?) But the foods that have been good for your body have been good for your body for hundreds of thousands of years.

That's exactly why I call myself the Primitive Health and Fitness Expert: Your body has the wisdom to know what's good for it. What's good for your body has been good since we were called homo sapiens. By and large, science has done very little to reveal a new miracle food or pill that wasn't known to be good for us for thousands of years.

Let's take on a few of the things pop-culture nutritionists promote that you should be very skeptical about now.

Low-fat, Low-calorie

Oh boy! I could write an entire book on this one. Didn't we learn our lesson in the 90's with the low-fat craze. These two trends in weight loss led to more problems than benefits, like poor bone density and women who couldn't get their periods on crazy, low-fat diets, etc.

Let me prove my point by starting at the end– the result of decades of the low-fat, low-calorie nonsense. Years into the obesity crisis we're experiencing, most women come to my practice and want to lose weight. Yet they come in saying the following:

"I will skip meals and eat less food, because eating is the reason I'm FAT. I know that calories are the reason you gain weight, so I'm going to eat less."

This mentality makes my eyes turn red with anger. This is the hot garbage that's the result of decades of confused experts, terrible studies, and a complete misunderstanding of calories, movement, and how to be a lean, healthy person.

There is nothing further from the truth. I will tell you later why calories should never be your focus in weight loss. Even though I believe nutritionists have their heart in the right place, many of them are victims of thinking inside the box.

At a scientific level, do you lose weight when you run a calorie deficit? (burning more calories than you consume) Yes. But calories are not something you need to understand or follow as a person trying to lose weight. At no point in time did we ever have to count calories to be lean. They might be the true scientific reason you lose weight, but is this honestly the most important tool for you?

I will argue NO. Do you think we used to track calories when we were hunter-gatherers? Or for that matter, when we were hard-working farmers? Absolutely not. There was no box on the side of a chicken to read how much protein and iron you were getting.

What's missing? What was the holy grail of weight loss that our ancestors all followed merely 100 years ago that had the general population slim and strong? We'll get to that later. Sorry, I can't jump the gun and give away all the secrets yet.

So why in the world do experts tell you to focus on low-calorie diets, or even worse, low-fat? Because, it's what they know. It's the limited lens they have used to understand how to lose weight. It works in a science project, so it must be the way to get you to lose weight.

Again, back to the **Nourishment** versus **Diet** debate, low-calorie is about **Diet**.

Telling you the consumer to eat a low-calorie diet is what has led to millions of young, reasonably fit girls (often with the appropriate amount of fat for their teenage years) to restrict their calories and become sick when all they need is to focus on exercise or playing (something we used to do when I was a kid) and food quality.

What's Wrong with Low-Fat Diets?

Even worse is the quest for low-fat dieting. Let me cover some basics.

Facts on Fat:

> » You HAVE to eat fat to burn fat– it's one of the three macronutrients, and to have a proper metabolism, you've got to consume fat

> » Fat, especially animal fat, was present in the diet of basically every human culture known to man as long as humans have been on this planet

> » Fat keeps your brain healthy, protects your skin, gives you necessary cholesterol, etc.

Hmmmm. That's weird. How is it that people were told to get off saturated fat, that it's bad for our heart, and we'll lose weight faster by slashing it? Again, the industry throws the consumer around year to year with "new scientific discoveries." But what's good for us has been a part of our diet for hundreds of thousands of years.

Too make matters worse, what did the fat-free proponents tell us to eat more of in the 90's? Here came the food and fat-loss industry to save the day with a myriad of weight loss foods— margarine, hydrogenated oil, artificial sweeteners, and extremely processed low-fat solutions for every food group. And for the love of God, nutritionists jumped on the bandwagon.

These low-fat advocates pushed us away from eating what we had eaten for THOUSANDS of years and replaced it with chemically created, over-processed foods.

Processed food is basically anything that doesn't look like it flew, walked, swam, or grew. Not all processed food is bad, but there are a few big problems with it. It tends to be loaded with salt for flavor, it has dyes and preservatives to give it shelf-life and look attractive, and it's very hard on the liver to process.

BUT, Didn't Low-Fat Make People Thinner?

<u>I suppose low-fat advocates would argue that many men and women got thinner on their diets. I can help you lose pounds on my new cardboard and lemonade diet too. Would you like to sign up</u>?

Lots of things can make you skinny. But as we'll discuss in

chapter #5, skinny isn't always healthy. And many of the women who got skinny this way have done real damage to their health.

The Food Guide Pyramid, Agro-Business, and Wheat-Based Grains

The next major recommendation came from a few sources, and many nutritionists lined up and backed what the food guide pyramid said, even when it went in the face of history.

You all remember the food pyramid. Junk foods are a small part of the triangle at the top. And a nice, wide base was sitting there at the bottom for your GRAINS. You were told to get something like 6-10 servings of grain per day.

The Agri-business has jumped on this bandwagon big time. In fact, it's fairly clear that the grain growing industry was there in the room when the food pyramid was created. <u>You were told that grains, especially wheat, should be the center of your diet because of economics, not health</u>.

How in the world nutritionists jumped on board with this is beyond me. Wheat is considered one of the biggest allergens in the modern era. There are entire diseases— severe gluten allergies and Celiac, and even issues around autism— that are linked to wheat.

And yet, grains were promoted as the center of our diet for heart health and weight loss. Are there good grains? Absolutely, and I'll talk about them later. But grains are also the base of foods that make weight loss nearly impossible for many Americans. Think cereal, pasta, bagels, muffins, etc. These are not your friend if you're trying to burn off fat.

Again, I'll take us back to history and natural wisdom. Grains were in the diet of many traditional and primitive cultures. But there were a few big differences.

- » They were only processed by being flattened, cut or ground by stone

- » They were eaten in their whole form for the most part

- » They were NOT in every processed food (there was no processed food)

- » Like most food, they were eaten seasonally. Some could be stored for a chunk of time, but they weren't necessarily available all year

Luckily I have seen many nutritionists and health experts backing off the grain bandwagon recently. But again, the weight-loss experts followed another short-term trend based on this new science and not historical wisdom.

Soy...the New Wonder Plant

Let's look at another great trend in the 90's. All of a sudden, we had found the miracle food. Vivre la SOY! Alas, we had met the ultimate super-plant, capable of making us free of that nasty meat stuff. It would solve all of our medical concerns.

I suppose, just like most foods that are the next great

cure, this came from a few scientific studies about soy and the benefits of phytoestrogen. And now 10 to 15 years later, there's a lot more concern than confidence over this little miracle plant. Perhaps it is great in some scientific studies, but was it meant to be processed and added to half the foods we eat? (For a long list of nasty health complications, including promotion of some cancers and tumors, thyroid problems and prevention of ovulation, go to www.westonaprice.org)

Another big problem with soy is frankly the amount we consume in modern times and the processing. Again, soy may be fine in the right state, like a reasonable amount of tofu, tempeh or miso soup, but it's not meant to be consumed in the quantity and quality that it is today.

Most of the soy you consume is in processed foods. The food industry has put soy in practically every processed food as soy isolates and other by-products, and it's basically a useless filler to make their science project food. Even if soy were good for you, there's no way this is the case when it's been snuck into everything you eat. I'm talking about soups, crackers, breads, baby formula and cereal. Basically anything in a package has soy in it.

My earthy friends helped drive this bandwagon too. When they deemed meat the enemy, which I'll tackle next, they made soy the base of their diet. Soy dogs, soy cheese, soy milk, soy brains. Oy vey.

This is just one more example of the painfully short-sighted nature of experts and trends. The food industry started to sneak soy into everything you eat because it's cheap to produce and makes a great margin financially. But they were thrilled when "health experts" deemed

soy the new wonder food! I'd watch out for any new wonder foods that our primitive ancestors wouldn't have consumed.

Eat Salad, Get Fat
The Dampness Problem

Dampness is a term used in Chinese medicine. Let me describe what dampness is in a way you'll understand. You eat a big bowl of ice cream, and then you notice more phlegm in your throat and sinus. Within 30 minutes, you feel really heavy in your gut; a wave of fatigue comes over your body and thoughts. Your mind and limbs feel heavier and maybe even cloudy.

This is dampness. It's nasty stuff. And unfortunately, tons of modern foods are damp producing. Foods like:

- » Cheese and dairy
- » Sugar
- » Wheat
- » Cold foods like ice-water
- » Salad and too much raw food in general.
- » Processed foods
- » Fried or greasy foods

When the average American goes on a diet (something you should never do), they say something like "I'm going to eat a lot more salad so I can lose weight." But this is really the last thing you should be doing. And most of the time, when someone starts trying to lose weight by eating salad, they're DRASTICALLY under eating. And that's a terrible way to burn fat healthfully.

Will salad make you fat like my title suggested? Not exactly. But there are a couple of important things to consider here. One is body type, two is season, and three is quantity.

Are you a very damp person? Do you have a fairly squishy body type? Do you feel very mentally or physically tired after eating? Do you eat too much food from the above list? Then going on a diet with a ton of cold, raw salads could be a big problem.

What season is it? There's a time of the year where raw salads are going to be easier to digest. In the height of summer when it's hot out and you're more active, you can get away with more raw food. Generally, eating with the seasons is a great way to meal plan.

Lastly, what quantity are you consuming? If you think you are going to get lean by consuming mostly salad, I think you're asking for trouble.

Eating warmer, nourishing foods like soups and stews are easier to digest and use less of the body's energy to process. The battle to START the fat burning process can be very difficult, particularly if you are relatively weak and have a lot of body fat. You'll make this process more difficult if you try to live on cold, raw foods.

Finally, if dampness is a major issue for you, we'll discuss the role of acupuncture treatment in your weight loss plan in chapter #9.

Chapter 3

Red Meat Is Bad for You, And Other Silly Lies They've Told You

I COULDN'T HELP MYSELF, I JUST had to make this into its own chapter. This is one of my absolute favorite subjects to discuss. I apologize ahead of time if I offend some people along the way. I plan to.

And if you still choose to live without animal protein at the end, I accept the fact that even though I feel very strongly about the importance of meat, some will choose not to eat it based on religious, spiritual, environmental or ethical reasons. That's a personal decision, and I respect that. Just don't tell everyone you know that it's "Healthy."

How My Environmental Friends Did You a Huge Disservice

Oh, my environmental friends, how you have done the American public a huge disservice. My major at the University of Maryland was Political Science, but my focus was environmental politics.

I COMPLETELY understand the environmental issues around meat. I was actually a vegetarian for two years for exactly this reason. It takes more land, you've got to grow crops to feed the animals, it takes more water, it has damaged parts of the landscape, the runoff is nasty, etc.

There are also ethical issues which are very real: The meat industry is often cruel and disgusting. I would never tell you to watch the videos from PETA or other environmental groups, because frankly, they haunt me.

So why in the world am I still a meat advocate you might ask?

<u>I will advocate until I'm blue in the face that we framed the issue WRONG</u>. As a result of the environmental and ethical concerns, people have made meat the enemy, and then spent the last 20 years trying to prove the point that meat is terrible for us.

Consequently, instead of using our power as consumers to DEMAND better farming, better environmental practices, and absolute intolerance of animal cruelty, we spent all our effort trying to prove that meat is bad and soy is the answer.

I am sorry. You can show me any video you would like, any study you would like, or any anecdotal evidence that you would like about how you felt better once you eliminated meat, and I will tell you I don't believe it-- and nor should you.

If Meat is Bad for Us Then...

If meat is bad for us, then as I said before, why did virtually every single tribe, community, culture, and people of this planet for the entire existence of homo sapiens consume meat?

And as I said before, I'm sure you could do some research and find one or two cultures that have not done so. But I will tell you that's the exception to the rule.

I don't know your stance on evolution, so if you don't buy it, skip this paragraph. The basic premise of evolution is that every species adapts to best suit its environment. So if that is the case, and virtually every human population consumed meat for the last 100,000 years, then there is 0% chance that it's bad for us.

And if pro-veg people want to argue this point, then they need to take it up with polar bears, eagles, and wild dogs too, because it must be bad for them also. And you should be out in the woods telling the wolf that he needs a colonic…because years of meat are stuck in his system because it's SOOO hard to digest (tongue in cheek).

Let's Look at Our Ancestors for a Moment

I'll just pick a time and group of people that I know fairly well to paint a picture. Native Americans inhabited this region for roughly 20,000 years. During that time, they lived as a mixture of hunter-gatherers and agriculturalists.

Just like our modern farmers, they grew some crops to sustain themselves. Corn, squash, and beans were three crops grown together that provided a lot of calories. Grains existed, but not in the prolific amount that we think of.

One of the foods they consumed would make 90's low-fat experts cry. Pemmican was a food often used in times of travel– a mixture of three equal parts– fat, dried and pounded berries, and dried and pounded meat.

But again, these people were lean and didn't suffer from the same diseases we do today. They consumed whatever walked, swam or flew at all times of the year. Buffalo, deer, birds, fish, and so on. They ate every part of the animal, including the organ meats, bone broth and animal fat. Many of them shaped their migration and lifestyle completely around the animals that they survived on.

I get very nostalgic about those times, as I believe there was a purity of life and purpose. They didn't confuse the sacrifice of animal for food as murder; it was respected. They understood that all life is sacrifice and that the plant gives as much up as the animal when you cut it from the life-cycle and eat it.

This connection is hard for us to understand today. Many laugh at this relationship. Others suggest that it is an over-romanticized picture of a very hard lifestyle. But no matter what your feelings are, it points out something pivotal to you and your understanding of fat-loss.

If you want to be lean and healthy, to live at the top of your potential, then you have to learn about nourishment. Animal protein is imperative for you to be healthy.

But I FELT so Much Better
When I Went Vegetarian

I've heard this one hundreds of times. Usually when I ask into it I come to one of two conclusions.

1. They are very new to vegetarian eating. Carbs and plants are much lighter energetically. If you live on plants primarily, you will indeed feel lighter in your body and mind for a while. There's a reason so many meditative communities stressed vegetarianism. It is conducive to leaving the body and mind. It makes it easier for you to feel light.

2. They used to eat terrible junk food and fast food. Then one day they went vegetarian. At that point, they started consuming a lot more fruits and vegetables, which will indeed make you feel a lot better, particularly if you've been living on junk.

But the problem with veg-only diets comes later down the road. And for every vegan who tells me they feel lighter, I've talked with ten former vegans who went back to meat and realized how vacuous, cold and tired they had gotten.

Over the long-haul, it is very hard to get everything you need without animal protein. Scientists at Weston A. Price have proven that you cannot get enough vitamin A, K, D and B12 if you forgo animal fat and protein. And while fruits, vegetables and some grains are great, you can't live to your fullest without meat. Secondly, losing weight without eating meat is a serious uphill battle.

In Chinese medicine there's a pattern called blood deficiency, and it's classic among long-term vegans and vegetarians. The symptoms of blood deficiency are:

> » Feeling cold internally— easily effected by cold weather

> » Dry skin and hair

> » Un-rooted thoughts and spirit (think mental clarity, or someone who seems a bit vacuous when you talk with them)

> » Numbness in limbs

> » Difficulty in getting pregnant and holding to term

Are there exceptions? Absolutely. Some people may be more suited for this diet, and some are just far more informed about how to do it successfully. But EVERY time I talk about my system in public a vegan or vegetarian has to get up and tell me that they've successfully gone without meat and they feel fine. Hey, there are people who've "successfully" smoked until they're 80 and they feel fine. Maybe you should take that up too.

I will tell you that it's very rare that I meet a vegetarian who is eating what they need to be healthy. Usually they depend on tons of pasta, processed wheat, and disgusting over-processed soy everything. Soy dogs, soy cheese, soy milk, etc. They will all tell you they get enough protein. I maintain they don't.

If you choose to be vegan or vegetarian for environmental, spiritual or animal rights reasons, I am fully in favor of you living in line with your beliefs. If you choose this diet, please do your best work to really learn about combining protein, and take the time to learn how to cook. You have a much harder job trying to get the protein that your body needs.

But if you choose to eat this way, stop trying to tell everyone how healthy it is. It's not. There's nothing in history to tell you this is natural so please stop taking the moral high road.

Before the Texan's Get all Hootin' and Hollerin'

MODERATION is still a reality. Let me just make two points before I am misunderstood: 1) I'm talking about really good quality meat. 2) I am not talking about a huge plate with a 20oz porterhouse and a side of potatoes.

If you are going to consider adding more animal products, you SHOULD listen to my earthy, meat eating friends. Quality is everything. The animal fat and protein our ancestors consumed was CLEAN.

It was not raised on soy or corn; it was not raised inside a huge, dirty factory building; it was not raised on chemically laden foods; and it was not given antibiotics and hormones or forced to fatten unnaturally.

I realize the price of really well raised animals is higher. But if you are going to add more animal fat/protein to your diet, you will not want to eat conventionally raised animals. If that's what you intend to consume, then I would caution you about eating more meat.

Thanks to consumer pressure and education, many more farmers are branching out and raising animals the way they are supposed to. Open pastures, outside in the sun, eating what they are meant to, and only medicating them when there is an actual need.

My family splits a quarter of a cow from a local grass-fed farm every year and keeps this meat in the freezer. You can quickly find a local source for grass-fed beef on the internet, and the price of buying in bulk like this is significantly better. We pay just $3.75/pound because we buy in bulk. It's best to buy it in the summer and fall when local cows (in colder areas) have been eating grass for months.

On the east coast, where I live, there isn't enough grass in the winter, so cow's live on grains. <u>Give them the months of spring and summer to live on grass again, and the amount of omega-3 in their fat will return to healthy levels</u>.

AND also, the quantity issue. I might be stressing the value of meat, but I am still talking about portions that are sane. Look at traditional animals. Most were very lean and had nowhere the amount of meat of a modern cow. People did not sit down to a 20oz porterhouse. And what you couple this meat with is half the battle too, so I'm not talking about a heaping pile of mashed potatoes as your vegetable.

In no way does this mean that you need animal protein in every meal, or even every day. I've had clients who want to add meat because they believe the health value, but they really don't want meat more than a few times a week. That can be absolutely acceptable if you just don't like it. You can take it more as "something your body needs" than something you love. I personally need it every day to feel mentally clear and energetic, but you'll have to find that balance for yourself.

CHAPTER #4

THE 39 MINUTE PRIMITIVE NOURISHMENT PHILOSOPHY

IN THIS CHAPTER, I'LL CLARIFY the system and theory around how you can use traditional wisdom to be the leanest, healthiest person you're capable of being.

Thanks to regulators, I cannot propose that you try any specific eating plan that I'm teaching. I am only allowed, as a licensed Acupuncturist and personal trainer, to suggest that you look at food differently. Thus, think of my advice here more as coaching or philosophy. I'm offering a different way to look at food. If you want to change your eating habits, I'm supposed to ask you to get told so by a doctor, nutritionist or dietician. Hopefully you'll have a doc or nutritionist that is open to new (traditional) thinking around diet and not modern goofiness.

I will also say that these same regulators protect the food industry to no end. I am not allowed to tell you to eat more grass-fed beef and colorful vegetables, but big industry is welcome to feed you pink slime, dye, pesticides (neurotoxin), etc. Another atrocity of the industry EXPOSED.

What I can promise is that I will show you exactly how you can become lean and healthy. I will show you a very simple path to melting body fat and being super lean. When you follow these principles, along with the fitness habits in chapter 7, you will find it almost impossible to hold onto excess body fat.

Do You Trust Your Body?

Bob Duggan, one of the founders of Tai Sophia Institute where I got my Master of Acupuncture, says something that is so simple, yet out of the ordinary for modern medicine:

"Your body is wise."

Does that sound entirely too simple to have any use for you? I hope not, because our current mentality around medicine and health is that your body is stupid. Do you have a pain? Take drugs to turn the pain off. Do you have a bad back? Cut into it. Basically, if something is broke, you need to FIX it.

Fixing a problem sounds pretty reasonable except that you run the risk of separating from your own healing and your own internal wisdom. Modern mentality around the body is much like someone who won't take care of their car properly.

If the engine light goes off, do you put duct tape over it? If the muffler begins to pump out too much smoke, should you just knock it off your car? This is the same thing you're doing when you cover up your symptoms.

What Does This Have to do With Nourishment?

For far too many people, eating has very little to do with nourishment. It's more like turning the "Hungry" button off in your body by stuffing your stomach with whatever you can find, or whatever you think tastes good.

What I want you to do is start thinking like "your body is wise." That you should learn what your body is asking for, practice different techniques around sleep, hydration, and eating that are more suited towards giving the body what it needs than stuffing it full to turn the "Hungry" button off.

Another word for the wise– following what "tastes" good has gotten us fat and sick as a culture. They can make almost anything taste good in a Petri dish, and then stuff it in your food to mimic natural flavors. If you currently eat a heavily processed diet, there will be a transition period where you will need to test your own taste buds to try new foods.

Much like a 5 year old trying new things, you will probably kick and scream a bit. Just think of yourself as growing up around food. Think of it as expanding your pallet so that you can be a healthy person.

Eat like a Lean Person, Not like a Heavy Person Trying to Lose Weight

I said this before, but I feel the need to say it again. Do you want to be a lean person, or a heavy person, perpetually working to be skinny?

If you're answer is the former, to be a lean person, then shift your focus and think like a lean person. Notice I'm saying "LEAN" person and not skinny. There are a lot of skinny, unhealthy people. Everything I'll cover below is my suggestion for how you can live like a lean person, even if you are 50 or 100 lbs over weight. If you couple this with the fitness principles I'll cover in chapter 7, there should be no reason you will hold on to excess body fat.

Are there faster ways to lose weight? Yup. You are welcome to bang your head against the counter, forcing down boring, low-calorie and low-fat meals. You will probably drop body fat, muscle, and yes, pounds very quickly.

But will it last? Rarely, if ever. In fact, they've created an entire category for this type of weight loss– the Yo-Yo Diet.

In short, here's what happens. You eat fewer calories than you burn, you burn body fat (and usually lean muscle). Your weight drops, but because you lost lean muscle, so too did your metabolism.

THEN, you get bored of the diet, because it's probably as fun as eating cardboard for every meal. And my guess is that you're not eating enough meat on this diet. So the second you get sick of the diet and run right back to your high-carb craving foods, you balloon right back to your original weight. Even worse, you probably get even heavier because you have lost muscle too.

Drag this out over 15 years, like many women do, and you've got a hormonal and digestive system that's a wreck.

The 39 Minute Primitive Nourishment Plan

If you follow the system I've created with my **39 Minute Primitive Nourishment Plan**, you can expect to drop around 1-3lbs of body fat per week. But because you are doing this by consuming the best foods, and at the same time as you're building lean muscle, you'll see so many positive changes, it won't matter how fast the pounds come off.

The fact is, they will come off. I have met maybe 1 in 100 people who seemingly follow the plan to a "T" and can't lose weight. This usually is explained to a trip to their doctor and a diagnosis of a legitimate thyroid disorder. I say legitimate, because this is the new fad diagnosis that everyone who doesn't lose weight uses as an excuse. "Oh, I can't lose weight because I've got a thyroid problem," or "I've got bad genetics."

For a small portion of women, they truly need to be on thyroid medications to get their numbers right. Once they find a balance with their doctor and get back on our plan, pounds are able to come off appropriately.

So read through this section, and then couple this with the exercise plan in chapter 7. I'll wrap the movement and nourishment plan up in the final chapter in an easy to follow way so it's not too confusing.

Junky, Processed Carbs are THE Issue

Not meat, not fat, not calories or eating too much. Junky, processed carbs are THE big issue.

Let's take a look at our ancestors again. Most hunter-gatherer populations did not practice agriculture, meaning they had almost no exposure to grains. It's only been in the last 10,000 years that some populations grew and harvested grain. For a fascinating take on this transformation in human population, read my favorite book of all time, <u>Ishmael</u> by Daniel Quinn.

But nowhere in time have we ever consumed the amount and poor quality of carbohydrates as we do today. If you don't really know what a carb is, think sugar.

The average American diet is a roller coaster of carbohydrate highs and lows. Cereal and juice for breakfast, a sandwich on bread with chips or soda on the side for lunch. Pasta with a loaf of bread on the side for dinner. Maybe four to six sodas or other sugary drinks during the day.

In short, you will find it IMPOSSIBLE to lose body fat and be healthy if this is the way you are eating. Your body is going through a roller coaster of blood sugar spikes and drops that it cannot handle. Then pop-culture tells you to cut back on meat, and you're making matters even worse.

I will work to give you a wider range of options at the end of this chapter, but for now, here's the NO list:

>   Juices and sodas

>   Bread, pasta, most cereal and other processed grains

» Candy

» High Fructose Corn Syrup

» Partially Hydrogenated Oil

Back to Our Ancestors

Equatorial cultures had more high sugar fruits (ie. Banana, mango, pineapple), and colder areas tended to have more low-sugar fruits (ie. Blueberries and apples in North America).

Grains were consumed. Quinoa, rice, barley, and millet for example. But there were some big differences to the way we consume these foods now.

First, what seasons were they consumed? Rice might have been available year round, but in colder climates, grains were tougher to keep during a long winter. So grains were more available in certain seasons.

Second, processing. You would have eaten grain boiled, ground by stone, or some other basic form of cooking. Modern bread is very different. Wheat (especially Gluten) is blamed for many modern diseases from Celiac to irritable bowel, to emotional disorders.

Because of its ability to make bread rise, and to make things like muffins stick better, wheat is more and more processed in modern foods so that it has a feel and taste that we like. This level of processing has made a perfectly useful carbohydrate from grains, into an over-consumed, highly inflammatory, allergy producing food. Third, amount. We just didn't have access to this food in the amount we do today. If you eat bread, pasta, cereal, muffins, and crackers every day of your life, you are getting very high doses of highly processed carbohydrates and gluten.

And that's not even counting ALL the other sugars in our diet today. Again, if you eat processed foods every day, you are getting a ton of sugar in your diet. The food companies are onto this, and they know that the consumer is more informed today, so they've worked to hide sugar from you in food labels.

They now have a list of over 100 different names for "sugar" in processed foods. <u>And they all do the same thing to you and your blood sugar. If you want to lose weight, you've got to manage blood sugar spikes. You cannot lose body fat successfully eating from the list of sugars, over-processed grains, and drinks like juice and soda</u>.

If it Didn't Walk, Fly, Swim or Grow, Don't Eat It

Processed foods are the second biggest concern. Maybe in terms of health they are really number one.

This one is really simple. Like the title says, if it didn't walk, fly, swim or grow, it's processed. Are their exceptions? Sure. Do you need to avoid all processed foods to be lean and healthy? Nope.

But the important thing here is the amount and quality. I'll often have clients put unsweetened rice or almond milk in their smoothies for breakfast. That is processed, but it doesn't worry me like other foods. I'm also a fan of high quality supplements (yes, processed) for reasons I'll explain later.

Some of the most common processed foods people eat: Chicken nuggets, or any other food where they've essentially mashed together "stuff" into a shape and fried it (news flash, much of your nugget isn't even meat); all bread products (muffins, bagels, etc.); candy; artificial sweeteners; and canned soups with tons of chemicals in them.

From a Chinese medical perspective, if your body doesn't recognize the "food" you're putting into it, and you're living off processed foods, your stomach and small intestine have to fight and figure out what to do with it.

Your stomach finds it tough to convert this food into something useful, and your small intestine is unable to separate the good from the bad parts for digestion and elimination. So the body can't make energy out of it, it can't absorb it correctly, and you can't live healthfully off it. This, again, leads to excess fat storage and health problems.

Fat Doesn't Make You Fat

I think people imagine fat gain this way. Eat meat and fat, it goes into your stomach to be processed, then it takes a direct train right to your love handles. Sorry, but no. That process is a lot more likely to happen with too many carbs (sugars) than with a reasonable amount of good fat.

There's a reason there's three macronutrients: Protein,

fat, and carbohydrates. Somehow fat got the bad rap in the 90's. Give me a break. Our ancestors cooked with animal fat for god's sake, and again, unless you don't believe in evolution, every species adapts to best suit our environment. We, as humans, did so by consuming animal fat and protein consistently.

Fat will not make you fat if you live off the healthy kinds. Sources like grass-fed beef, nuts, and avocados are great sources.

Did I just say red meat is "Good Fat?" Absolutely, if the cows are fed the proper diet and raised without hormones and other unnecessary drugs. In fact, grass-fed beef is actually high in Omega-3 fatty acids, the healthy stuff you're told to get from salmon.

If you look for grass-fed beef in the grocery store, you'll find that it's very expensive. I want you to still consider eating great quality beef, so like I said before, look up some local farms who you can buy from.

I know this is all tough stuff to wrap your head around. Eat some fat, eat meat. Sounds so very confusing. But please go back to where I started. The fat-loss and food industry has been putting out crazy information to the public for decades. Their number one goal is profit, not your health. Most of what they say is based on product sales and crops they can grow for the best margin, not the stuff that makes you lean.

The Four Keys to all Good Food Choices

More than any point system, calorie counting system or

fad diet, following these four simple steps will get you lean. And the beauty is these aren't that hard to follow.

1. Easily Digestible Foods

2. Frequent Meals/snacks

3. With the Season

4. Frequent Protein

I promise, consistent application of these four rules will send you in the right direction quickly if you truly follow them.

1. **Easily Digestible Foods**– This partly refers back to the dampness issue that I discussed in the second chapter. Choosing digestible food means food that's quickly transformed and absorbed by your stomach. It means foods that don't increase dampness and inflammation (eg. Foods that increase dampness in particular are dairy, sugar, and wheat).

I remember the first time I went to a wilderness survival camp. Every day, the same boring food. Oatmeal in the morning, and soup for lunch and dinner. And the soup was literally just broth, rough cut veggies, and meat.

I saw a transformation in my body within three days. THREE DAYS! My stomach went flat (mostly from bloating I was carrying), my skin got firmer all over my entire body, and I fit in my pants differently by the end of the week.

Now I am not proposing you eat like this, because it's boring and you'll never sustain it. But there is wisdom in the simplicity here that you should learn from. Eating an easily digestible diet devoid of inflammatory foods will make weight loss and reduction in bloating VERY RAPID.

So what constitutes as easily digestible?

» Soups and stews

» Basically all cooked veggies (maybe excluding white potato)

» Fruit in its whole form (not juice or processed with extra sugar)

» **Unprocessed foods– Processed foods require that your body work a lot harder to extract anything useful**

» Lean meat (remember– don't believe the anti-meat propaganda)

Use this list as a starting point for looking at your diet/ nutrition. This is in no way a nutrition guide or a cookbook, but I'm trying to build the case for wise practices that will promote rapid fat loss, and easily digestible is a good start.

2. **Frequent Meals/Snacks**– People I respect differ on this one. There's research to prove that we need times of fasting (even a day with just fruit or tea). There's research to prove that frequent meals and snacks is the best way to be lean.

Here's my take on this whole issue. I know it might sound strange, but there is a good case for short, scheduled times of fasting if you look at our ancestors. BUT, this is one time where I will contradict my own promotion of

Primitive Wisdom. The role of fasting might have held up better in a traditional culture where 1) people were already lean and 2) people didn't have the level of stress that we deal with today.

I've even tried some of the nourishment plans that involve times of fasting, and most of them left me feeling tired and brain dead. They just didn't work. They did encourage a quick change in my gut (reduction in belly bloating), and I had improvement in some of my primary symptoms (like heartburn), but it was just too tough to sustain.

If you're reading this book, most likely you've got some pounds to lose. I'm convinced that the BEST way to do this is through frequent, smaller meals and snacks. In **39 Minute Workout**, all of our clients who've had success have adopted the four principles above, and FREQUENCY is a big one.

Tame the Wave

The value of frequency is like a bell curve. Think of the top of the curve as blood sugar spikes. The bottom is blood sugar crashes. If you follow an eating plan that has you up and down that severely, like most Americans eat, you will have a heck of a time losing weight.

One of the most important ways to turn ON your Primitive Fat Burn is eating food with reasonable frequency. Something like three meals and two snacks is a good target. By getting consistent whole food and good protein, as I'll describe in the fourth tip, you'll tell your body to go into fat burn mode. And that's the

whole point. You're either storing or burning fat, and frequency is key.

Picture this wave in an analogy around emotions. You always want to live in the middle, small range of emotion. Too high is mania, too low is depression. If you live somewhere in the middle, and can keep this level of balance (with the 3 Pillars that I am teaching) you will have good health, good relationships, and a good quality of life.

But if you choose to live at the extremes, whether with blood sugar or emotions, life kinda sucks. Everything is too extreme. Too up, too down, never happy.

This is the way you should view weight loss. If you can keep your emotions and blood sugar steady, you will lose weight much more easily. So **Frequency** is one of the powerful ways to ensure just that.

Keep the body steadily fed every two to four hours at the most, and you will help keep your body in that middle zone. That perfect, comfortable zone in the middle is where your health can flourish. For me, it's four good sized meals. For some, it's three meals and two snacks. You've got to find the food and frequency that produces results.

3. **With the Season: A brief lesson in Chinese medicine**– We have the ability to get any food, whenever we want it. And sometimes that's really nice. It's great to have bananas all year round, and oats, and rice and so on.

But you want to think with your primitive roots like I've encouraged. The food that grows in a specific season isn't an accident. The season in which I'm writing this book, for example, is spring. What's coming up at this point? Small greens that are pungent like scallions and arugula.

In Chinese medicine, there are five seasons, and each one has two organs associated with it. The spring for example, is called the Wood element (think growth of plants), and its Organs (Chinese medicine set of attributes, not the actual organ) are the Liver and Gallbladder. The spring is about rising energy, new plans, vision for your year to come, and taking action on what matters most to you.

Your body has specific needs in this season. You've just come off a long, probably more sedentary season where you ate heavier foods and got outside less. The liver needs to get moving, as do your muscles and sinews. So it's appropriate to get outside and stretch your muscles out again, to get more vigorous in your exercise, and to make new plans for the year.

Going back to the foods of the season, these bitter herbs that are available in spring help to cleanse the liver, which is the organ that processes and stores toxins. Going with the knowledge of the season, if you consume the foods that the earth provides, you will benefit your health.

If you want to live at your best potential, to be lean and vibrant, eating with and understanding the season is very appropriate. Notice that there's more fresh fruit and vegetables available in spring and summer. There are more dark greens, root vegetables and legumes in fall and winter. Follow what's appropriate for the season, and you will find better health, because your body will be getting what it needs when you need it.

This also takes care of another need. We need a diversity of foods for good health. If you get in a rut and eat the same foods all year, you're less likely to get the full range of nutrients that you need. So eat with the season and promote great health.

4. **Frequent Protein–** It happens very often when I speak to a prospective client. I ask them what they're doing to lose weight and they happily tell me they've stopped eating red meat. Yikes! Not a good way to start your fat burn.

Most of the food journals we see in our practice have a couple of big flaws that keep people from losing weight. One of the big ones (besides very infrequent meals), is lacking quality protein in meal after meal. We've seen people go days with no more protein than a small cup of yogurt.

Here's a little secret about our ancestors. When they had access to meat (and animal fat), in general, they were doing well. Our bodies, over thousands of years, adapted to this reality. If meat was plentiful, it was a time of success. If we were living off of carbs mostly, we were in a time of struggle.

Imagine a tribe following caribou around the landscape. They tracked these animals for hundreds of miles. There were times that these animals were elusive, or their numbers dwindled because of die off from food shortage or natural disasters.

When the animal numbers dwindled or the tribe simply couldn't get access to them, their health struggled too. They lived off of foods that lacked fat and protein. For their bodies to handle this time the body adapted for survival.

What do you think your body will do more easily in a time of success? What do you think it will do in a time of struggle? You can probably guess, in times of success, the body doesn't need to store fat as much. Times were good, and reserves of fat in your body weren't as dire. But when animal fat and protein was sparse or non-existent, the body was forced to <u>store</u> whatever it could.

This is the second key to turning your Primitive Fat Burn ON, besides frequency. You have to consume good amounts of animal protein to burn fat. Skip out on it, and you'll depend too much on over-processed carbohydrates. Eat enough, and you'll help turn your fat burn on.

So again, if you are trying to lose weight by cutting down on meat, which many of the "experts" in the fat loss industry are telling you, then you are going against thousands of years of evolutionary wisdom.

When our primitive ancestors went without meat and animal fat they struggled to get the nourishment they needed. Their bodies literally started to consume muscle. But you live in a time of abundant food, so when you go without protein, you most likely reach for poor quality, nutrient lacking foods.

Most of what I see is that people who skip out on healthy protein over-consume junky carbs. They grab fast energy food in the form of chips, deserts, and other sugar or wheat based foods. So instead of getting the protein they need to feel satiated, they grab cheap energy foods that pack on body fat.

This then feeds the cycle of fat gain. You eat foods that spike blood sugar and your body stores fat. If you want to promote your Primitive Fat Burn, you've got to eat protein with regular consistency.

Don't Tell Your Husband, but I Encourage You to Cheat

On your nourishment plan that is! You didn't think I was getting into love advice too, did you?

Why completely avoiding your favorite foods will lead you to fail...

I will introduce this concept and explain why I believe most people should cheat on their nourishment plan. But I always pose this thought to my clients in the beginning of our weight loss challenge, if eating some of your favorite "cheat" foods will take the stress out of it, then have some. If cheating some will lead to cheating a ton, then this tip is not for you.

You've got to know your personality and be honest with yourself. You've got to know who you are. Are you all or nothing? If you have one bowl of Ben and Jerry's, does it quickly become one pint? If that's you, you may not want to cheat.

This came from my own exploration with nutrition. When I got really serious about food several years back, I went on a very strict meal plan. I have no more control than any of my clients; I just tend to shop better. I am just as much of a fan of a good burger or ice cream as anyone else. I think that's what makes me a good trainer, because I don't have these superior feelings of, "Oh if you just lived on celery and did sit-ups for breakfast you could look like me."

No, I struggle with food discipline just like you. So when I got more serious about following the nourishment plan that matches my values and would promote my optimal health, I had to create a plan to deal with food cravings.

I decided that if I could cheat on the weekend, then it would be easier to tell my brain it's not forever. We live in a world with a lot of great tasting stuff, and a lot of it isn't good for us. But if I could have one day that I had access to whatever I wanted, then I would have more self-control during the week.

Years later, this technique still works for me, and it works for many of my clients who've had success. But as I said, you've got to know who you are. Many of my clients cannot go there. They are all or nothing, so a brownie on Saturday will lead to the donut at work on Monday, and the bagel on Wednesday, and the beer on Thursday. So for them, it's all or nothing.

If you are this type of person, the cheat day is not for you—at least not until you reach a goal. We'll talk a lot more about setting goals and carrying through with them in chapter 8, but for now, decide whether you need to cheat to have control during the week, or whether one cheat will destroy all your good effort. And BE HONEST.

I Don't Like Water, Oxygen, or Going to the Bathroom

Three equally ridiculous claims. So WHY is the first one so common?

That's what I hear all the time. If water is yucky to you, I will say two things. One, you probably have a ton of dampness. Go back to the list of damp foods (sugar, cheese, milk and wheat) and eliminate them to see how you feel.

If you live off of them, you've probably got a ton of dampness, and what I find is that damp client's hate water...until I get them to back way off their damp foods or get them some acupuncture. We'll cover the role of treatment in chapter 9, but if you have really bad dampness, acupuncture will speed up your healing a lot faster than diet alone.

Two, get over it. "I don't like oxygen." "I don't like going to the bathroom." Those statements make about as much sense as saying you don't like water. So why would you say this?

Your body is made of water. Take ten minutes and read all that water does for you and your health and you will be unable to defend skipping it. Mental clarity, energy level, emotional balance, performance in sport and work. And that's not even all the hard science around your cell function, ability to detoxify, and a litany of other stuff that water is a primary player in.

If your goal is to be lean and healthy, you cannot go without good amounts of water. And do not let yourself think you can get enough by getting it through tea, coffee, soda or fake water substitutes. If you really want to drink other things too, at least have enough water every morning to pee clear by 10am. That's actually one of my weight loss rules that you should follow. I know, really technical isn't it?

I read a blog once from a well meaning nutritionist. I think she should lose her certification for it.

She was making a case that we don't have to work so hard to drink water every day. She said you can get water from vegetables, and that the old misnomer about coffee counting against your water consumption was bogus. That there's enough water in coffee to count towards your total, and caffeine barely makes you lose water.

Project: Please do this for one day (tongue-in-cheek). Drink only coffee, and eat a ton of celery. The next day, I'd like you to drink enough water to pee clear by 10am, and then once again by 3pm. Then tell me which day you are more mentally clear, physically aware, and emotionally happy.

She is certainly correct that you get water in your veggies. But if I know the average American diet, you are not getting nearly enough veggies. And the fact is, most Americans are dehydrated on a daily basis based on their trips to the bathroom. If you go hours without needing to pee, and every time you do it's dark, you are not drinking enough.

And the fact is the list of benefits from water is too long to cover in this book. And the negatives are non-existent. You would have to work really hard to over-drink water.

I'm not sure it would be possible, but maybe if you had gallons you would stress your kidney. You would have to work hard to do this.

Actual Project: Follow my water rule for two weeks and pay particular attention to several things— bloating in your belly, energy level around 3pm, and mental clarity through your work day. You will be amazed. If you made daily notes in a journal before and during this project, you would see some great changes.

The Most Overlooked, Slightly Mundane, But Absolutely Crucial Habit for Health

Just like skipping meals, it's shocking how many people say they don't sleep well. This has to cost us all in terms of poor energy, higher stress levels, and lower productivity at work. Long-term sleep problems are also linked to higher levels of obesity and heart disease among other health concerns.

There are really two categories of people here. One are people that do everything right and still don't sleep well. This could mean you think too much in bed, have bad dreams, have sleep apnea because of actual sinus problems like a deviated septum, or something else completely out of your control.

For this group, you need to read chapter 9, and learn how acupuncture can help you.

So what are your sleep habits like? Do you have good sleep hygiene?

Here's a simple checklist:

» Do you get into bed after 10:30pm?

» Do you read or watch TV in bed?

» Do you need some form of sound distraction to put you to sleep?

» Do you need medications or alcohol to get to sleep?

» Do you give yourself at least 8 hours of sleep?

If you've checked any of these bullets, then at least part of the issue for you is poor sleep habits. And part of getting a good night's sleep is giving yourself a chance to get a good night sleep. So if you're someone that stays up past 11 watching TV or "being productive" as many say, then you're biting into one of your most basic needs.

Let's look at our ancestors again. In general, they followed the sun cycle. They didn't have light bulbs and interesting late-night TV. They didn't stay up late at night to get work done.

But here's the reality about our body. It doesn't care about your preferences. It believes you should follow the sun cycle, so if you don't, it suffers. It is built for more sleep in the winter, and less in the summer.

You might describe yourself as a night person, but that's more of an addiction. That's what you've gotten used to. I promise that your body is hard wired not to believe you or thrive under those circumstances.

I actually find that most people don't give themselves nearly enough time to sleep. Many people only allow for 6 hours or less, go to bed later than 11pm, and/or get up too early. They often site that they are productive late, they enjoy being up, or it's the only quality time they have with their partner.

Many of these reasons are valid. It's really tough if you're in a relationship and this is the only time you see your partner uninterrupted. But if sleep habits are making it hard for you to be healthy, you might need to create some boundaries or practices that can help.

The problem with sleep as it pertains to weight loss and stress is important. I haven't gone into hormone levels much. They're a little out of the scope of the Primitive Health and Fitness world, but they are a major factor in weight loss and healthy aging.

People are suffering from many hormonal issues these days. Many clients come to me for acupuncture presenting with these hormonal issues. Thyroid disorders, low testosterone, adrenal exhaustion, menopause, and high cortisol levels to name some of the most common.

Although you don't necessarily need to understand hormone levels, suffice it to say that your lifestyle will directly help or hinder you when it comes to balancing them. And good nutrition, quality sleep, alternative therapy, and consistent exercise are the four most powerful non-drug ways to control these symptoms from above.

Your sleep habits can either set you up for health, or create an uphill battle. So it's extremely important in your quest to be lean and young that you set yourself up with good habits. Here's a short list to support you:

» Give yourself at least an 8 hour window to sleep

» Get in bed before 10:30pm

» Don't eat any later than 2 hours before bed

» Don't consume caffeine after 12pm

» Go to bed before you fall asleep on the couch

» Provide yourself with a "wind down" routine that gets you in bedtime mode

This is by no means an exhaustive list, but it's a good start. The point I want to stress here is that your long-term health and weight are very closely linked to how much rest you get. Rest also impacts your daily energy levels for working out, staying motivated and positive, and making good food choices. And like learning, trying to cram in rest over the weekend will not support long-term health.

The Primitive Health and Fitness Nourishment Plan Summary:

1. **Eat Frequent Meals**—from 3-5 meals a day, eat until you're full, fill up with the right stuff and you'll burn fat like crazy

2. **Eat Good Amounts of Protein**—How much? Don't worry about grams. Just get a good quality protein in each meal. Add some sort of fiber, like bean, to stay full too. Coupling the two will help you stay satiated…the key to fighting cravings

3. **Eat Unprocessed Food**—Eat food that looks like it came from the ground or was once alive. This will mostly ensure you keep with low-glycemic

foods. The key is to eat foods in their natural state

4. **Eat with the Season for good variety!**

5. **Drink tons of water and keep peeing clear**. Remember, only hard-science here

That's It! Could you go into more detail? Sure, but it's probably too much info. Just follow the rules, enjoy your once a week cheat day, and watch the pounds burn off. And chances are, you need to be eating a lot more food than you are today. Most of our female clients under-eat and have destroyed their metabolism. This will be a change to actually FILL UP on healthy foods. No diets here.

PILLAR TWO

TRAINING

CHAPTER #5

RICE CAKES, DIET COKE, AND THE HAMSTER WHEEL

T RAVEL IN TIME WITH ME. We're in a huge, crowded gym in the late 90's. Hundreds of skinny, "healthy" women are on a sea of fitness machines. They're pumping their body's into a sweaty fury on the treadmill, stair-stepper, and elliptical.

They sip from their water bottles like hamsters on the wheel, and read their favorite trashy mag while they "enjoy" their exercise. Or maybe they watch their favorite program on one of the 20 TV's above the machines.

After a nice hour and a half of cardio, Jane hops off her machine and heads to the strength circuit to hit a few of her favorites. Maybe she even does some presses or bicep curls with some appropriate 5lb pink dumbbells.

Now back home for a light lunch. Rice cakes and some

light yogurt, and of course, some diet Coke to wash it down. She has to keep her calories low, and she only ever eats low-fat foods of course.

Who Else Wants to Spend Their Entire Life in the Gym?

I didn't think so. Then I would not emulate Jane.

We'll talk about how healthy Jane is on her insides later. But for now, let's look at her exercise habits, because they're being followed by THOUSANDS of well meaning women trying to lose weight and stay "healthy".

It's assumed because Jane is so skinny, that we should follow her habits. Do what she does. Pick her machines and follow her routine. Let me tell you a little bit about Jane's routine, because it's still the routine of choice for most women, and it's making your success almost impossible.

Jane picks routines that are "appropriate" for a woman:

> » Very light weights
>
> » Long-boring cardio
>
> » Lot's of FUN classes— I'll skip naming them so I don't offend too many people
>
> » Five days a week or more
>
> » Described as fun and easy, never strenuous

Let me be clear, I'm all about routines being fun. They should be. But if you don't want to spend your life working out, then there are some big problems with these routines pitched to women.

Let's take these bullets one at a time.

Women Should Lift Tiny Weights???

Let's look at Jane's choice in weights now...and have another history lesson.

Women are told to use machines and do light isolation moves with very small weights to get lean muscles that look feminine. Ok, do you know where muscle isolation came from? That's right, from people who have the body every woman would love to have– **BODY BUILDERS**. Ummmm. Excuse me?

Yes, muscle isolation is a technique that came from body building. It doesn't make your body move better, it doesn't give you better bone density or help you burn more fat. It quite simply gives the muscle a pump.

This is much like western medicine. It looks at the body like the sum of its parts. If you've got a few hundred muscles, how many isolation exercises would it take to "Get Fit"? More than you have time for.

Muscle isolation is taking one muscle, like the bicep, and doing a motion like a curl to target it. There's nothing implicitly wrong with muscle isolation, but there are a few problems, number one being that it will take forever to get you fit and firm, and it will have much less impact on your metabolism.

That means that you'll have to spend a ton of time working out if you choose isolation. And if you're like my female clients, you'd like to be firm in your butt, upper arms and core. Let's talk about how to quickly get you a firm butt, arms and core.

Where in the world did this notion come from that women should lift light weights? I've got children. Do they feel light to carry? Does it feel light to carry luggage? Do you think our primitive females were weak and lifted only 5lb things?

Women may not have the same ability for maximum strength that a guy has, but that does not mean she's supposed to be too weak to pick up luggage without back and shoulder pain. Or to have to ask a man to open a jar of pickles for her. Or to carry her son while she's making dinner with the other arm.

The concept that women are supposed to life light weights came from a very false notion that they will end up bulky like a man.

In my practice, I've seen how this works. All my ladies lift "heavy" (appropriately heavy for them, and a lot heavier than they first imagined when they walked in the door). And at the most, one in a few hundred women can actually build muscle of any size.

If that is you, you probably already know this. And even if you are that one in a hundred, you still should lift weights. There are simple ways to make sure you burn off any muscle size if you don't want it, and it's the same thing a guy would do to keep lean muscle without bulk.

I'll tell you what I did with the one client I ever had who could build bulky muscle. We capped her weights at a certain number (no presses or kettlebell swings over X lbs). We stressed longer sets, and she's supposed to focus more on muscle endurance and cardio instead of heavy work in our classes.

The moral of the story— IF YOU AREN'T THAT 1% OF WOMEN, THEN YOU CANNOT BUILD BULK NO MATTER HOW HARD YOU TRY. SO GET A TRAINER AND LEARN HOW TO LIFT HEAVIER.

Why? Thanks for asking.

Well, we both agreed that you'd like to burn fat efficiently, spend less time in the gym, and get firm where you want it— particularly upper arms, core and butt.

This demo is more powerful in person, but I think you'll get it. Imagine I stand and press a 5lb weight overhead. Now I pick up a 35lb and I press. Which one do you think will make my arm harder? Of course it's the heavier one.

If you want to firm a muscle, it would benefit you to make it harder when you train. So if a heavier weight will make your muscle harder, it will also "store" that tension in the muscle well after training a lot more efficiently than that little paperweight.

My female clients might do 25 presses with an 18lb kettlebell in a class. And they have great arms. If you opt out for the "safer" pink weight, how many reps and how much time would you have to do to get the same result? Way, way, way too long. And frankly, it may never build the same level of appropriate strength you need for life.

"I lift Light Weight's because they're SAFER"

Pardon me for my bluntness, but this mentality comes from our excessively soft, pampered culture that's gotten entirely too far away from the primitive bodies we still live in.

Who do you think has a better back and bone density? Our primitive ancestors. They carried heavy things and they sat on the ground and had to maintain good posture instead of slumping in cushy seats all day among other things.

As I write this, a common large gym chain has a really funny commercial. This muscle-head is taking a tour of the gym, and he keeps repeating "I pick up heavy things and put them down." All the while, Barbie and Ken dolls are in the background happily using a myriad of machines.

The funny thing is, you've got more chance of looking like a muscle head by "getting a pump" on a machine or with a free-weight. You're better off picking up heavy things and putting them down.

So let's talk about safety. It's so common that people think heavy is unsafe. But that's the mentality of a culture that's takes gym class out of schools, allows all our weak kids to sit in front of the TV all day, and suffers from endless back problems.

It is not only safe to lift heavy, it is actually a liability to go through life never lifting heavy things. Your muscles, joints, sinews and bones are all designed to endure stress. They need you to lift heavy things, to use your body, and to pick up heavy things and carry them.

People who go through life not wanting to lift heavy are the ones that suffer from bad backs, weak cores, sore shoulders, and they usually age terribly when they hit their 50's.

If you never pick up something heavy, your back never develops the strength to hold you up correctly. Your shoulders never develop the muscle to hold together correctly, so you strain them by doing something simple, like picking up your child. You see this in people who age and can't do simple things like climb steps, carry groceries, or stand up straight.

Again, as is typical in our culture, the blame is in the wrong place. We should fear weakness and slothness, not heavy weight. We should fear the chemicals in our food, not eating animal fat. I don't know how these cultural norms develop, but in this case, they're not keeping you safer.

A Word of Warning

Before you go start a routine where you lift heavy, let me make a recommendation. If you have pain or limitations in normal, everyday movements, or have a prior injury, you need to get checked out. Whether by a trainer who can do a Functional Movement Screen (FMS), an acupuncturist, a Physical Therapist, or doctor, you need to get pain taken care of before you lift heavy.

While I do believe you need to lift heavy, at least as part of your routine, you've got to do it safely. Pain is a funny thing. Keep working out with pain, and you'll set yourself back. You've got to get into a routine at an appropriate pace for your age and athletic ability.

So before you get started, think about finding a trainer

like the ones on our staff who can do an FMS and help you identify any red flags.

I Want to Lose Weight I'm Going to do More Cardio

I hear this comment from people wanting to burn body fat all the time, and it's a major misnomer. Depends on what your definition of cardio is. Are you talking steady-state cardio or intense intervals?

Let's look at Jane's favorite choice. She was a child of the 70's, so she got fit starting in the 80's when aerobics was all the rage. Scrunchy socks, headbands, and yes, beautiful print or pastel lycra outfits.

This, along with any class that has you dancing, pumping, or riding a machine at basically ONE level of intensity for an hour or longer is steady-state cardio, EVEN IF YOU SWEAT A LOT OR "FEEL" LIKE YOU'RE WORKING HARD. Another hallmark of steady-state is that you never get over about a 5 with intensity. So there's no real sense of strain or explosion of effort.

To clarify before I make you too mad, any of the above workouts can be made into a useful type of cardio and fat loss routine. I'll show you how in Chapter 7.

There are so many reasons women have been told to work out like this. People assume intense workouts are dangerous. They assume intensity means muscle growth. And maybe it's because getting over a 5 makes you scared. It shouldn't. It's all about using a system that makes sense and having a trainer that knows what the heck they're doing.

But here's the big issue I have with all these fun workouts being pitched to women: They're painfully long and pointless. They do nothing to build lean muscle, nothing to work the heart the way it really needs, and they burn fat so inefficiently it's almost pointless.

If you look at this from a traditional perspective, we might have walked long distances at times, but most of the work we did was strenuous, like carrying heavy water containers up a hill (now that's cardio– try it).

The issue with your common "fun cardio" class is the efficiency. Because they don't use weights that are challenging enough, and the intensity never get's high enough, you burn very little fat and you have to work forever to make any changes to your physique.

I actually love the Biggest Loser for a few reasons. One of them is this exact reason. You see the most obese, unhealthy and often un-athletic people busting their ass with weights and machines, and they burn a ton of fat.

You are probably not nearly as bad off at Biggest Loser contestants, so you are completely able to handle intense workouts. And you will reach your goal a lot faster. Yes, they do some steady-state cardio, often when they workout alone, but when you see them with the trainers, they're huffing and puffing, and putting out an 8 or more with intensity.

117 or 450?

If I gave you a choice, how many minutes would you like to train every week? Unless you REALLY enjoy the gym,

I'm guessing you'd prefer 117. My weight loss clients train 3 times a week for 39 minutes, and they have great results.

If you'd prefer the slow cardio and light weight workout, give yourself more like 90 minutes five times a week to get the same results. So again, in terms of doing more "cardio" to lose weight, you've got to ask what kind of cardio.

If you're picking classes because they're fun, but nobody is losing weight, and it takes an hour or more to get done, I promise you it's not what you should be focusing on if your goal is weight loss, increasing bone density or changing your body tone in minimal time.

If you have a class that you love because it's fun and you love the community, then keep doing it. It's great you're moving. But please find a way to get some weights and intensity into your workout at least two days a week. It will go a long way to improve your results.

Jane the Gym Nut– From the Inside

Jane is obsessed with her weight. Her body is what every woman would describe as "perfect," but for Jane, it's never enough. She lives in the gym, eats a steadily controlled diet of less than 1200 calories, consumes very low fat and very little meat.

Jane was the inspiration of this chapter. She's operating under all the status-quo beliefs that the fat loss industry and common trainers have promoted. In their eyes, she's doing a great job.

But Jane has a few issues we should discuss. She's under consumed food so long, she lacks the fat she needs to develop strong hormones, so when she hits menopause, it's brutal. Crazy hot flashes, and energy levels that plummet frequently. Her memory is slower, and her skin and hair don't have the vibrancy she once had.

Jane was a Barbie doll on the outside, but after years of training and eating like this she's paying the price for eating too little and working out too much. Her bones are thin because she never lifted heavy weights, and she never got the fat and nutrients she needed from her practically vegetarian diet.

The Chinese have a saying, and Jane lived her life in this way. You can cheat your health until 30. After that, your health will cheat you.

But I don't get it. Jane did everything right by modern standards. If you've read everything so far, you can tell me exactly why this has happened. It's no secret that Jane did not feed the needs of the primitive body she lives in.

You can live to fit today's standards of what a woman should look like, but I would suggest you do this by following the primitive rules that will get you there safely. There are way too many Janes after the last few decades of diet craziness.

And no, not all beautiful, slender women are sick on the inside. It's all about how you get there.

CHAPTER #6:

RIPPED AND WORN OUT⃞ THE 90 DAY PLAN TO ADRENAL EXHAUSTION

I'VE JUST SPENT A CHAPTER talking about all the workouts that are way too light and inefficient to get you results. But now, there's a new beast to contend with on the market too.

At first glance, you'd think I'm saying the same things as this new beast. They stress intensity and weights. They give you a system to follow, stress low-carbs, and push you to be your best.

But just like the bell curve I described with nutrition, there's a curve with exercise too. The last chapter was all about workouts that live at the bottom of the curve.

Now there's a breed of psychotic, hormone crashing

workouts that live WAY AT THE TOP OF THE CURVE. I'm talking about workouts that go at an 8 intensity or above, up to six days a week, and incorporate moves that are only designed for high-level athletes, and should never be done on a long-term basis.

They are the new "wonder pill." The magic solution to make everyone ripped and looking like the models they usher out, and they have great before-and-after's to show you. "Look how good this worked!"

Ok. I see your pretty models. Let's have them do your workout for six months and we'll check in on them physically and emotionally. And let's see some really heavy, out of shape and un-athletic people do these routines for more than three weeks without injury. Then I'll be more impressed.

My 2,168 mile Story of Mental and Physical Exhaustion

Let me tell you a story. It's the story of the most powerful experience of my life. If you read my intro, you've already heard a bit about my hike. But now I'll tell the other side.

From April 2 to September 30, 2001, I hiked the entire Appalachian train from Georgia to Maine. I already told you what a powerful experience this was. It was highly spiritual for me. It helped me evolve, and I believe it set me up for the jump into my new career in health.

But there's another story too. It's the story of what this hike did to me physically and emotionally. I was not lying when I told you this was the most powerful experience of my life and that I'd do it again in a heartbeat if I had time.

But it was also a great sacrifice. It took a toll on me physically. During the hike, I suffered with painful plantar fasciitis for over two months. I struggled with tons of heartburn in the middle states.

When I got to Connecticut, there was a day when I was practically flying up the side of a mountain. I had just passed a family of day-hikers, and I was cruising up this steep slope when my legs felt like they'd been dropped in cement. For the next two weeks hiking was painful and slow. Every bit of stretching, days off in Vermont, Epsom salts baths and effort I took to alleviate this new, sudden drop in performance was futile.

Thank God my legs came back in New Hampshire right before the most difficult portion of the trail in the White Mountains. Then the last month, my sweat took on a new smell as the last of my body fat stores were burned off. I don't want to describe the smell, but let's say it was tough to put that shirt back on in the mornings at that point.

Afterwards, my knees were sore for over a month. It hurt to walk down steps, I was depressed for at least four months afterwards. That fall I also experienced the worst allergies of my life.

The acupuncture treatment I received in those early post-hike months was the only thing that helped me climb out of it.

Why in the world am I sharing this story? Because this is what happens to the body when you over-train—

when you take on a workout claiming to push you to your very end of intensity. I did this as a personal accomplishment, a race against myself, an experience. I did not hike the trail to get healthy.

What happened to me physically and emotionally was very hard to dig out from under. <u>Would you like to do a workout that will promote physical and emotional collapses like I had to deal with? Then do not train like this</u>.

I would be very leery of a program that has you busting your ass at crazy high intensity for over an hour a day and up to six days a week. This has the look and feel of exactly what I did to myself. You cannot endure that kind of intensity for long before there are costs.

The only time I believe this intensity is appropriate is with a personal challenge like a marathon, hiking the Appalachian Trail, or training for something like the Olympics. But in any of these cases, you're not doing them to be healthy. Most people who run a marathon can tell you they don't feel "healthy" afterwards.

Your intention for working out is about a different type of accomplishment. It's taking your body to a place of firmness and leanness that you've never had, or never been able to maintain. It's reclaiming your health, not crashing it.

Once you get to the point where you're at your goal weight and you've maintained this health for over six months, then consider taking on some personal challenges. I've noticed that when my female clients get near their goal weight, they get the itch for physical accomplishment.

People find it deeply satisfying for all kinds of reasons to meet new goals or complete challenges they've always dreamed of.

Many have sought out adventure races, 5 and 10k's, and even marathons. That's great. But do it after you've built a base of strength and lost a lot of weight. And do it for the right reason…accomplishment. Not because you saw this killer workout on TV and everyone looks ripped!

Busy Work is NOT Training

What's your goal? Is it to spend a ton of time in the gym or a workout program? Is it to look and feel like you're BUSY?

I hope not. But that's what so many programs do.

Look, just because a workout feels busy, feels challenging, doesn't mean it's accomplishing much. And it sure doesn't mean it's getting you closer to your goal.

You can join any number of programs on the market today and FEEL like you're getting a lot done. But when you break them down— how long do they take, are people in the class getting results, are they teaching nutrition, etc.— they are just busy work.

It would be very easy for me to just wear you out. I could run you through a busy work program that FEELS like it's really hard, you would be worn out at the end and feel like you got a lot out of it, and get ZERO results.

WHAT! How can that be?

There are two big reasons: 1) Your primitive response

to excessive hard work/stress is to put the STOP sign on weight loss. 2) There's no progression of skills– are you working out or training?

Let's break these two ideas out in more detail, because it's very important that you get these concepts before you create a plan to lose weight and be healthy.

The STOP Sign on Weight Loss

There are two big ways to put the STOP sign on weight loss, and just with everything else in this book, they both have roots in your Primitive body.

I described the first one in my chapters on nutrition. Under-eat, or don't eat enough animal protein, and you struggle. The result is that you will reach for low-nutrient, junky carb foods that put on pounds.

The other way to turn off fat loss is to constantly bust your ass in vigorous workouts that are hard for long periods of time. It's exactly what I described in my Appalachian Trail experience, and some of these new 90-day wonder workouts.

But frankly, there are a myriad of new workout routines on the market. Many of them are emulating each other. Their focus: bust your ass until you're a puddle on the floor. Result: you feel like you've worked really hard. Lots of sweat was lost, soreness ensues, pat oneself on the back.

Sorry, that's not what your body is saying. If you keep this up and do this week after week, you end up just like Jane the gym nut from the last chapter. Even though she got there with crazy long, wimpy workouts and under-eating, you're going to get there for a different reason.

Remember, wear whatever clothes you like and use as much technology as you like, you are a PRIMITIVE being, and your body follows the same Primitive knowledge from hundreds of thousands of years of adaptation to our environment.

When do you think humans were stressed day after day like all these "BUSY" workouts? Rarely if ever. And if they were, like in a time of war or forced migration, their bodies would have suffered just like mine did on the trail and yours will in these workouts.

Do you think you'd go buy a copy of these videos if they were called **The Forced Migration Workout**. Or **90DayAdrenalFailure**! I doubt it.

The point of the story here. If your workout is too much like busy work, and if it's too many hours for too many days at too high intensity, you're doing more harm than good, and you're telling your Primitive body to shut down fat loss.

Before you Blast me Because They Get Great Results

I'm sure if you love these workouts you're saying "hold on, you can lose a ton of fat with them." Let me tell you the problem here. First off, men are much more likely to have success in workouts like this because we have more muscle and we'll burn fat through working out alone. Very few women's body's work like this. But for men, you have to worry about long-term adrenal exhaustion and collapse of testosterone...and you won't see that for a while, so it's assumed the workout is safe. I would disagree.

For women, let me tell you my point through a client of mine we'll call Jody. She came to us with about 20lbs to lose. If you looked at her you might think she had a few pounds to lose, but she was in no means far away from her goal.

She was in boot camps and other workouts SIX days a week. They were the type I've been describing here. Lots of busy work, long workouts, and yes, six days a week. The problem was that her weight loss had stalled.

My recommendation was to STOP working out so much. She joined our groups for three days a week, and stopped the other busy-work boot camp. She followed a few of my nutrition guidelines in our weight loss challenge (she's now in her second challenge– working to burn the last few pounds because she's very committed and consistent). And as I just suggested, she lost weight.

Even though she'd been in boot camps six days a week for years, she was not losing weight. I told her to do LESS??? I told her to eat more, but eat the right stuff. And the result– she lost about 15lbs of the 20 that she wanted to lose. And I can tell you that the last 10-15 are the hardest, so this was a real accomplishment. She just keeps plugging along week after week, because she values her health and she's committed. She is now doing LESS and burning MORE. She's doing it by following my Primitive solution to weight loss.

Plyometrics– A Two-Step Plan
for Blown out Knees

Step one, load your muscles with a ton of tension. Step two, jump and land with a ton of force. Step three, drop to the ground in pain…you just blew your ACL out!

Plyometrics was designed as a highly specialized program for Russian athletes. Want to hear a minor detail about them from someone who knows what he's talking about, Pavel.

"I shall wrap up the plyometric section by repeating the point that you must have a base of absolute strength before going explosive. And those levels are quite high. The Russian admonition not to start intense plyometric training until you can back squat a barbell equal to 150% to 200% of your bodyweight should give you a clue." (Easy Strength. John and Pavel, 2011)"

So unless you can squat 2X your bodyweight, and unless you can squat, butt to the floor with perfect form, and unless you have great glute strength (like from a kettlebell swing), you have NO BUSINESS doing plyometrics.

I am not insulting my clients when I say that most of them are not athletes and cannot do simple movements with proper form when they start with us. It's just the reality. They were never taught to squat correctly in gym class. They are usually carrying extra weight and they've been out of exercise for a while– that's why they've come to us.

And my clientele is no different than the average American. So why in the hell would products sold to millions of Americans use a program that's dangerous for the average person? I have no idea. Ask them.

For now, I'll tell you this. My clients who think they are squatting well, because they learned from a gym trainer… usually do not. Most lack any glute (butt) strength because that's a tough muscle group to work (and no, most runners don't use their butt much when they run). Most cannot keep their knees in line with their toes. And almost nobody comes in and can squat to the ground with the proper, tall posture.

We'll explain in the next chapter how I use progression to get all of my clients squatting well. It just takes some time and some proper drills.

So here's a scenario. Jenny the gym nut thinks she's in fairly good shape. She's got about 10lbs to lose, she does spinning at the gym, and she'd like a new program. She starts on one of these insane workouts, extolling the value of plyometrics.

Jenny doesn't know it, but she has poor hip mobility, so she can't squat down and load her hips with the proper tension. To compensate, she shifts her weight onto her toes and ahead of her knees. Also, each time she puts any real weight down into her knees, her left one buckles in. Her trainer at the gym had limited experience with correcting form, so he never taught her how to fix all of this.

So she gets her videos in the mail, and it's time to get pumped. She's going to get in the best shape of her life. Two weeks in, she's doing all sorts of explosive movements that involve jumping and fast lunges. Remember, each time she does this her form caves forward on both knees and inside on her left knee.

That week she feels a little pain inside her left knee but she waves it off. It's just the cost of getting a great body. What she doesn't know is that her body is giving her signals that she's moving incorrectly. Each explosive rep is putting unneeded stress on her body. By week three, there's also an ache in her low back down the left side of her butt.

On week four, Jenny really does it. In the middle of a mind-numbing workout, 40 minutes in, her body is getting overly fatigued. Her form is suffering, but Jenny is a work-horse. She's not going to stop just because she's a little tired.

Then it happens. One last explosive jump, form is sloppy, body is tired, and she lands really badly on that knee. She was at a fatigued point where her already bad form was even worse, and she tears her ACL. On the floor in significant pain, she's probably blaming her shoes. Maybe they didn't have enough cushion anymore.

But the problem was long before she tore her tendon. Jenny didn't have her squat form down. She lacked the strength in her support muscles, ankles and hips to jump safely. She had never been taught to squat with good posture using her hips and butt. She also had never even built the strength to squat 40lbs, let alone twice her bodyweight, so plyometrics was a questionable choice in the first place.

So whose fault is it? Jenny's for doing this routine? Her former trainer who didn't know how to teach her a good squat? The people who wrote these programs for the masses which are suited for high-level athletes with a great base of strength and form? Yup, all of them.

I don't want you to end up like Jenny. So PLEASE, before you start routines like this, you've got to get your strength, mobility and stamina ready for them. Learn from a program like the **39 Minute Workout** that teaches you a base of skills and progressions. Then follow our routine, and make your primitive body into the sleek, firm, and fit figure that you're capable of creating.

Chapter #7

Primitive Fitness Secrets From a 9 Year Old Apache Girl

How a Native American survivalist woke me up to our Actual physical limitations

WHEN I WAS AN INSTRUCTOR at the camp for troubled boys in Georgia, I read a lot of books from a survivalist, Tom Brown Jr. For years as I lived in the woods of Georgia, and then during my six month hike of the Appalachian Trail, I imagined being a character in his books. They were amazing tales of adventure, spirituality, and the primitive way.

Finally, after three years of acupuncture school, I went to my first class at Tom's school in the Pine Barrens of New

Jersey. This powerful, intimidating man stood in front of us for many classes and spoke about survival, of how we lived for thousands of years, and what we are capable of as humans.

Particularly, he showed me how small our limitations actually are. He showed that our perceived limitations physically, mentally, and in our senses were nowhere near our actual potential.

One of his comments stuck with me even though it seemed very subtle and unimportant at the time. He said, "A 9 year old Apache girl could carry more than you all." Ok, no big deal. Except he wasn't kidding. He was speaking to the fact that we were once much stronger and more willing to take on physical challenge than we are today.

Maybe we don't need 9 year old girls to be as strong as an Apache. Maybe you don't need to be either. But what he's pointing out is that we've become WAY too soft. We have spent too much time sitting on cushy chairs for long hours, staring at computer screens and TV's.

I absolutely agree with him. Every week at **39 Minute Workout**, I watch people come in the door because they are suffering. They've put on too many pounds, their health is suffering, they've got emotional challenges that are making life less pleasant, and they are looking for a way out.

When I talk with people who are in their late 40's and on, they start to talk about a reality that makes them very nervous. Many of them aren't talking about having a beach body, or getting a better butt. They are watching their parents getting older and losing function. They are watching what a life of never lifting weights does to mobility and ultimately to quality of life in later years.

This is a very real, grim reality for many people getting older. The way out is getting back to our roots; back to our primitive capabilities. That way is to get physically strong and lean again, and to give our body's the movement and nourishment that it needs to thrive.

I'm not implying that you need to have incredible strength. I doubt that matters to many of you. But you would like to carry groceries or luggage without pain. You'd like to be able to pick up your kids, mow the lawn, play sports, and age well with good bone density and muscle strength that will help you maintain a happy and more independent quality of life in later years.

In the rest of this chapter, I'll discuss the plan to get you to live at your full capability. I'll introduce my **39 Minute Workout Primitive Movement Plan**.

But first, I've gt a bone to pick, and it's with our doctors and other professionals.

Helpful Doctors (and other Professionals) Put the STOP on Success

I am not going to mince words here, because this one really gets in my craw. We have gotten to be serious babies when it comes to our bodies and exercise. And professionals are not doing anything to help our cause.

We've turned our world into a padded, painfully "safe" boring place where we're scared of real exercise and weight but we embrace the lazy.

I don't know where this comes from, but I've witnessed it over and over when my clients tell me about advice from doctors, physical therapists, chiropractors, and other professionals. The professional meets a client of mine for two seconds, hears two words about some ache or pain the client's dealing with, then on a tiny piece of information, here it comes: "I'd recommend you stop that workout and do a routine with light weights...or easy cardio. That's more appropriate for you."

We've had countless clients who have finally gotten into a routine that is shedding body fat, helping them be more mobile, getting stronger bone density, feeling happier in their lives, and working out consistently for the first time in their lives.

Then they hit a speed bump. Maybe their hip gets a little sore, or their neck or arm, or whatever. They go to their doctor, tell them they've got a stiff this or that, and here it comes. The doctor doesn't ask any more questions like:

- » How long have you had this pain?

- » Did you have it earlier in life?

- » Is it better or worse with movement?

- » What has improved in your life because of this program?

Nope. No more questions. Just "it hurts here." Then doc says, "Oh, you should stop doing that program." As a personal trainer and licensed acupuncturist, this drives me absolutely crazy. It reminds me of the phrase **don't throw the baby out with the bathwater**.

I think it comes from the fact that so many doctors feel

compelled to always give a diagnosis. So they come up with some ten cent theory and tell the client to stop the ONE THING that's gotten them to the best health of their life.

<u>And hey, if you're coming to me to drop 50lbs and, as your doctor recommended, to get your high blood pressure down to a safe level so you don't stroke out and die, then I think that supersedes a little back stiffness. I find that in most cases, you can move through your back stiffness if you work with me, communicate, and give it time. But if you just quit and do that "safe" routine at the local gym, you'll probably stay at that same weight. So you have a choice, work through your back pain with me and stop being a stroke waiting to happen, or listen to your gun shy doc and stop the routine.</u>

One time I called my Physical Therapist friend, Kelly Sykes, and said, "What the heck do PT's have against kettelbells?" He laughed and said, "Nothing." We discussed for 15 minutes, the role of doing basic movements like kettelbell swings and squats to strengthen the back and core, and how our ancestors didn't have the back problems we have because they used their core all the time, didn't sit on cushy chairs, and they were strong. We both share the same philosophy that proper exercise with appropriately heavy weight is great for back health, and that's how primitive people had strong backs and cores in the first place.

And from this discussion, I realized yet again, that many professionals will make snap judgments that are way too conservative when it comes to the body. So before you go to your doctor to get your body pain checked out, or to ask her if kettlebells are safe for you, make sure they know what the heck they're talking about. If they've never heard of a kettlebell swing, don't ask them. They'll hear the words "swing a ball of iron between your legs while bending your waist" and say not to do it.

They aren't in my classes watching 66 year old women doing kettlebell swings with perfect form, dropping 15 lbs and gaining bone density. They aren't there to watch us take countless people from a history of bad backs to "0" pain in a matter of weeks.

***If you do genuinely have a physical limitation or pain, get it checked out. Find out if it's something serious (like a ruptured disc or torn shoulder cuff), or if it's nothing that shows up on an x-ray. If you're cleared and you still have limitations or pain, that's what trainers are there for.

We work with people that have pain every day. I've had thousands of people who've come to our classes with a history of back pain, shoulder problems, etc. And in most cases we're able to guide them through the process of getting a strong core (80% of the issue) and work through it. Having pain is not a reason to skip an excellent strength and fitness program like ours. It's merely something that has to be worked through with trained professionals that have dealt with this hundreds of times.

Do not opt out for a "safer routine with light cardio and light weights," because as I'll demonstrate, that's a load of crap. You are that same human as the 9 year old Apache. You aren't built for pink dumbbells.

Alright, let's get down to it.

The <u>39 Minute Workout</u>
Primitive Movement Plan

Step 1: Pick up heavy things and put them down

Have you seen the commercial for Planet Fitness? I love it.

Huge guy with foreign accent taking a tour of the gym. He keeps stupidly repeating, "I pick up heavy things and put them down." Everyone in the back is happily working out on their machines. They look like beautiful and happy Barbie and Ken dolls, and here's this muscle-head sticking out like a sore thumb. The Planet Fitness employee secretly escorts him out the back door and shuts it behind him.

The scenario they create is certainly funny, but here's what I find most humorous. Although he's a goofy muscle-head, what he's saying makes a lot more sense than what everyone behind him is doing.

What do you think is more natural to us as humans? Sitting on a machine, strapping your leg in, and extending your leg over and over to "get a pump," OR picking up heavy things and putting them down?

I think the answer is clear. Want to know the other funny part? You have more chance of looking like that muscle-head by getting a pump on a fitness machine than by picking up heavy things and putting them down. Heavy does not make bulk, getting a pump does.

Our primitive ancestors had the same needs that we do today. Let me repeat that in a different way. Our needs haven't changed in well over 100,000 years. And as humans, we're built to pick up and carry heavy things, press things overhead, and pull things towards us. There are a few other basic movements but not that many. Maybe add a rotation like throwing, then running and jumping, and you've basically got all your needs taken care of.

So when these modern fitness studios want to act all superior with their 10,000 machines and good looking models posing in the background, I would take it with a grain of salt. They are not offering you the movement that your body needs or wants! I would actually pay a lot more attention to a workout that has you "pick up heavy things and put them down."

Here's a list of appropriate lifts that fit that bill:

>> Front Squat

>> Farmer's carry

>> Kettlebell swing/Deadlift

Why do you NEED to do these lifts?

>> They work up to ¾ of all your muscles in one motion (that's how it's 39 minutes; it's efficient)

>> They help you build a strong core—key to a good back

>> They are basic movements to all humans—if you want to age gracefully and get through all your life's needs, you need to do them

>> Doing these movements with weight is the best way to build bone density

And a few more words on your core. How do you think

our primitive ancestors worked their core? Did they get on the dirt and do their crunches? I'm sure you know the answer by now. They picked up heavy things and put them down.

If you learn how to appropriately do the list of three exercises from above, you will build a very strong back and core. Do this safely and progressively, and you'll see amazing changes in your back health.

Please, as with all my advice, don't go and do this stuff unless you know what you're doing. Most of the clients who come to **39 Minute Workout** cannot squat correctly when they start. And almost nobody is teaching the kettlebell swing correctly (God help Biggest Loser contestants!), so please don't try this one without a properly trained instructor. Chances are that you already do farmers carry. Just carry two armloads of heavy groceries, with your arms straight at your side, and you've got the idea. It is worth getting with a trainer to learn these basic movements though. So go get trained on a proper squat at the very least.

Now get out and listen to that muscle-head. He had it right!

Step 2: Explosive lifts for stronger heart, bones and butt!

Why ALL Women Have to lift Weights

Sounds crazy I know. But if you want to have a strong heart, strong bones, and a butt that defies gravity, the second step of Primitive Fitness is imperative.

Remember back to my chapter on women lifting tiny weights? I told you it takes a ton of time to get you results, will do very little to make you more firm where you want it, and it will do almost nothing to build good bones.

So what in the world do I mean by explosive? Snappy, fast, powerful, etc.

There's a huge list of explosive exercises, and many aren't safe for you. Powerlifts and plyometrics (without proper training) are the two that come to mind.

Frankly, I'd put sprinting and running into that category for most people too. Far too many people are taking years off their body by running or sprinting with too much body weight, terrible form, or a very weak body. Done wrong, explosive lifts will just cause injury. This really draws into the content from the last paragraph. High rep jumps with bad form.

But!!! As I like to say, don't throw the baby out with the bathwater. There are some excellent explosive workouts out there. And the single best one is the kettlebell swing.

Done correctly, under an RKC trainer at our **39 Minute Workout**, the kettlebell swing is the single most efficient, fat-burning, bone-building, butt lifting exercise there is. And it's a very safe explosive lift under the right trainer.

Here's exactly why you need to incorporate this exercise into the core of any good fitness and fat burning routine.

People Watch too Many Dinosaur Movies– The key to Primitive Heart Building

I've heard this hilarious argument from some doctors and trainers. Basically it goes like this. "We aren't designed for long, steady-state cardio. We are designed for short bursts of energy, like running away from a tiger."

I TOTALLY agree with one of these assertions. We are designed to get intense bursts of energy, and that is how we got to be so lean and strong as primitive people. If you don't believe me, I've got a task for you. I'd like you to grab one of those three gallon buckets for painting, run down to the closest river or stream, and then carry that beast back to your house.

That, my friend, is not steady state cardio. That is one butt whooping exercise that will get all your muscles working, your core strong, and your heart pounding like a drum. You are built to do this, and much of the primitive work was VERY intense cardio.

But the other half is a little funny and oversimplified, and I think too many of these experts watched bad dinosaur movies where people were running from sabertooths. Ummm. Not too realistic. We are just about the slowest animals out there, so if we were only built for sprinting away from animals, God must have made us as a joke, because we aren't outrunning any predator.

My point is just this. We are absolutely designed for short bursts of work. But we are also designed for long steady-state work too, like hiking around the landscape in search of plants, water, and animals. We migrated, we hunted and gathered.

This way of life required a good mixture of very intense work, like carrying water and wood, or tanning hides and building shelter. But it also allowed for long walks and other peaceful cardio that had us lean and healthy.

Our ancestors didn't study the newest scientific "proof" or studies on their heart. They didn't follow trends or the next great diet. They simply lived, and their life gave them everything they needed to be healthy and live long, productive lives.

My conclusion: We need a good mixture of steady-state cardio AND intense intervals to have a healthy heart.

But we also need long cardio for other reasons. Things like challenging yoga, walking, running, biking, swimming, etc. There are emotional reasons you should be doing these exercises. Just like acupuncture, good slower, fun forms of cardio like these will help you de-stress, move lymph, move stagnation (see ch. 9), and so on.

But, as good as cardio is for reducing stress, it STINKS at burning fat. You should not be doing steady-state cardio to build a stronger heart or burn fat. That will take forever, and it will never build a firm lean body that functions well the way lifting kettlebells will.

So the **39 Minute Workout** Primitive Fitness Plan includes a mixture of high intensity and low intensity cardio. But I'll always put more stress on intense cardio for two reasons. One, this is the one most people lack or are unduly afraid of. Two, this is the one that will make the biggest impact on your physique and heart health.

Two Options for Better Bones

You've got two options to build better bones. I'll let you choose. You can get really heavy and walk around like that for the rest of your life, OR you can lift weights.

Great, I'm glad you chose the second option. Now let me share a story with you. Ellen joined our group when she was 66. She'd been working out with another trainer for years, since she turned 60, but when he moved out of town she thought she could do it on her own.

Over a year passed, and she had to come to the realization many people do. She was just not going to go to the gym or working out on her own. She wasn't going to be consistent, push hard enough, or know what to do.

She was also facing another issue that many women experience at her age. Her bone density was going down. She and her doctor were growing concerned, and Ellen really didn't want to go on one of the prescription drugs for bone density with a litany of nasty side effects.

So Ellen decided to join our classes. Within the first 6 months, she went back to her doctor to have another bone check, and to her shock and the doctors, she had gained 4.5% bone density!

Ellen is a very slight, thin lady who had never lifted weights or worked out her entire life until 60. Now, even at 66, she was able to re-build bone density by simply adding our **39 Minute Workout** classes and making very slight changes to her diet like eating more leafy greens. That's it. Two years later, and she's right there at basically the same levels. And she stays consistent with our classes.

Come watch her swing a 35lb kettlebell with no problem. You'll be in awe.

Why did our workout help her build stronger bones? She followed the first two principles of the **39 Minute** system. She picked up heavy things and she did explosive lifts. Explosive lifts do the same thing to the body as picking up heavy things. They put stress into the skeletal system and the bone responds by getting denser. Again, you can get overweight, or you can lift heavy things.

A Butt that Defies Gravity

I don't make "this is the best thing EVER" claims often… except when it comes to building a better butt and the kettlebell swing. Our client, Nancy, recently told us of a real life example to the amazing kettlebell butt.

She was laughing with some ladies in class, telling a story too quietly for me to hear. Then I caught wind of the fact that she'd been on a date recently, and the man was rather impressed with how firm her butt was.

Nancy came to us with about 50 pounds to lose. She has two grown children, and she wanted to get back into the dating scene with more confidence. She's now lost over 32 lbs and counting. When we asked her what she was most impressed by with her transformation, she said "for the first time in my life, I am an athlete!"

How about that. A 55-year-old woman feeling proud and describing herself as an athlete. And she's got the "kettelbell butt" to boot.

So if you don't know what a kettlebell swing looks like, take

5 minutes to watch my videos on <u>39minuteworkout.com</u>. When it's done correctly, the kettlebell swing requires you to bend at the waist, lengthen your hamstrings, and then tighten your butt really fast until you're standing. You're holding a weight with a handle with both hands, and your hips and butt are propelling it.

With every rep, your butt gets stronger and tighter. In less than 4 weeks, you should notice significant changes in how firm it is, and where it sits. Most clients lose inches in their waist within the first month and feel significant changes in their butt, core and arms too.

I don't care what machine, sport, or class you take. Nothing competes with the kettlebell swing when it comes to making a great butt!

There are other explosive lifts that we use in class, like the clean, clean and push press and low-impact jumps. They will all make improvements in the look and feel of your body. The key to explosive lifts is that they will do more to make you firm and burn fat than wussy workouts with tiny weights or endless cardio. If you want fast and significant changes to your butt, arms and core, explosive lifts need to be part of your repertoire.

Step 3: Frequency and Intensity

Quality Not Quantity

The man credited with bringing kettlebells to the United States, Pavel, always stresses to "leave one in the tank." He really opened my eyes to the value of doing all that your body needs, and not one rep more.

In an era where tons of sloppy reps are the norm, I find his perspective refreshing. And that's the way I've modeled my system. You've got to train within your limits and give your body what it needs. Nothing more.

So there are two keys to how hard you should work out: frequency and intensity.

In terms of frequency, I've already stated that six days a week of intense workouts is WAY too much and will simply lead to breakdown in your body, mind and health.

The answer to frequency depends somewhat on your goals, your other activities, and your age. I can't really say everything about the right frequency for you here, but our system can help you personalize the right amount for you.

If you've got significant weight to lose, like over 20 lbs, you need to work out a bare minimum of three days a week. I would recommend three or four days of intense **39 Minute Workouts**, followed by maybe one or two days of more relaxed movement like walking (vigorously), biking, etc. If you try to go too hard, you'll stop your weight loss. So never do more than four days of tough workouts in a week.

If you've got another sport that you love and do consistently, two or three days a week can be appropriate. I would never do less than two though. We've had serious runners in our groups, and they've all seen significant benefit to their sport with just two days a week of our sessions. They've developed stronger arms, core and stamina that translate to stronger running in just two days.

If you're over 55, you've got to pay special attention

to your limits. You will want two or three days a week, but you'll want to keep your intensity slightly lower than your younger classmates. As you age, you've got to find that intensity level and frequency that has you feeling stronger, and NEVER depleted. If you feel depleted after a workout, discuss this with a trainer. You probably need to dial down your intensity.

Walk that Fine Line

There's a fine line between INTENSE and BURNED OUT. You've got to find that line through trial and error, and that line will change depending on the season (yes, we're not built for the same output in the winter), stress level in your life, how well you're eating, etc.

I want our clients to work very hard. I want them to work at an intensity that most of them are not used to. That takes time and trust to get there, but the rewards are great. If you are willing to pick the right weights and work at an 8 or 9 intensity for short spurts with GREAT FORM, you will see the changes in your body and health very quickly.

But if I seem cautious, I am. I'm cautious for several reasons. Most of you will lack the core strength and body awareness at first to push really hard for an entire **39 Minute Workout**. You've got to give yourself 2-6 weeks depending on age, weight and athleticism to build up to great intensity. This process is, no doubt, best worked through with a trainer who knows what he's doing.

I have two rules in our classes that you need to follow religiously. 1) no back pain 2) no sloppy reps

If at any point you experience any pain, and I don't mean "damn this is hard," you need to stop working out and do some foam rolling, or switch up the exercise you're chosing. For example, a new client can't usually handle an entire class of swings like an experienced one. When their body starts to wear down, we'll have them use an easier exercise like jumping jacks or body weight squats. As I said about the professionals that will tell you to quit at the first site of pain, I'd say learn from it.

You have to be smart. If you get a twinge in your back, shoulder, knee, that's a warning. If you listen to the warning and stop your workout right away, most likely you'll be fine, and you'll be right back two days later. Choose to be a tough guy and push through it, and you'll probably end up truly hurt. Then it's weeks out of class, and that does no good.

So the rule of thumb with pain is to stop what you're doing and foam roll (Google "foam roll" if you're not sure what that means), or stop doing the one lift that's bothering you for that session, and get your form checked out.

Most pain is a result of bad form. This is why a certified trainer is so valuable. My staff and I can watch your swing, squat or press and fix what's wrong in several minutes. Usually it's that easy. So give your body the necessary weeks to build up to a good intensity, and keep focused on form.

That brings me to the second rule you've got to follow. Always lift with good form. There's a rash of Crossfit gyms out there doing some things that are good (explosive lifts, etc.), but they tend to value slop over quality reps.

This would never fly in our classes, and it shouldn't be a part of your workout. If you get to the point of some high intensity intervals and you feel that you just can't swing the kettlebell with good posture or you can't hip snap correctly, pick up your jump rope or choose a favorite callisthenic and continue. DO NOT continue to do bad reps just because you're tough. Tough people end up with injuries. If you're in a class and you experience excessive fatigue and your trainer tells you to keep pushing, quit now. That's stupid macho advice that gets people really hurt and run down.

Up next I'll discuss the difference between training and working out. This will do a lot to explain the value of exercising smart. Always keeping good form is the hallmark of training.

Are you **Working Out** or **Training?**

Training is a progression of skills. Working out can be anything– look busy for thirty minutes and break a sweat. Great, you're working out.

But what the heck are you accomplishing with working out? Often, very little.

The second problem with these hormone crashing workouts and many of the modern busy work workouts is that there's no progression of skills. They are workouts.

The characteristics of Working Out:

>> You look busy

>> You get a pump

» You break a sweat

» You feel tired or sore afterward

Whoopty Do! Remember, I said that constant hard work puts a STOP on weight loss. So does doing a workout that does not progress your skill. I'll explain why working out without developing more skill/athleticism will not progress your physical transformation.

These characteristics of working out above may make you feel like you're doing something, but they don't have a lot to do with weight loss, health, or progress. They are markers that show you very little. You can break a sweat every day of your life in some lame circuit and never lose a pound.

Let's compare that to Training:

» Learning a progression of skills

» Becoming more athletic– getting better at basic movements

» Moving with ease and experiencing less pain

» Being able to do something you couldn't do before

Unlike the list under working out, these skills under Training will ALL get you to where you want to go. If you're a 55 year old woman, you might scoff at the idea of being a better athlete. "I'm long past the days of caring about being an athlete," you might say.

I'll have to disagree. Would you like to be able to pick up your grandkids without pain, to play with them on the playground, to play tennis late into your life, or to travel with your husband, and do all this without physical restriction? Would you like to have the strength to get through life and never be held back by your body's limitations? Great, then you want to be athletic.

Progression of Skills

Simply, Progression of Skills looks like this, and again, I'll use a client story to explain. My client Sandy joined us almost two years ago. She was in her mid 60's, was maybe 50lbs overweight, had yo-yo dieted her whole life, and had really lost strength and function by the time she came to me.

When she started she literally couldn't get up and down from the ground without several minutes and assistance from someone else. She could not squat down and raise back up from a chair using only her body weight without assistance. She couldn't press overhead until her arm locked out, or do a basic kettlebell swing with safe form. This is an extreme case, but the end of the story (which isn't over because she's still training with us and still doing great) shows you the value of progression.

Over the first few months, all we worked on together was to get her good at basic movements that would benefit her life. If she couldn't squat or get up and down off the bed, imagine how her quality of life would be in 10 years. You squat every time you sit down, climb steps, pick something up. You may not think you care about a good squat, but hopefully you will after Sandy's story.

It was not an easy process, but together we got her squatting and swinging a kettlebell safely. To squat, I put a chair or a bench under her butt. All I wanted was to see her sit on it with good form (knees in line with and behind toes, hips bending, tall posture). For months she was rarely able to get down to the bench. Progress seemed slow at times.

Her swing was safe, but it wasn't long or explosive enough to be a great workout yet. I'll explain "explosive" in the next chapter. We had to get pounds off her belly and thighs while we worked on her form at the same time.

By that winter, her body was showing real change. People at the school where she taught were commenting on how good she looked. Her face, arms and belly were all showing the 28 pounds she'd lost.

Flash forward six months. Now she was able to squat down until her thighs were parallel with the ground, she could swing a heavier weight (makes cardio and fat-burn more productive), and she could get up and down off the ground in class! Up until then, I'd always had to adapt her workout to all standing exercises.

Sandy has been a client for over two years now. And here's her list of accomplishments:

- » Dropped over 30 lbs

- » Holds a true plank for up to 45 seconds

- » Gets up and down on the floor in 10 seconds

- » Squats with perfect posture, butt below her knees

- » Swings a 35 lb kettlebell!

How 'bout them apples? That's progression at work. If

she'd have just done a "fun" class where she sweat, she may very well never have gotten a stronger core, dropped the pounds, and she certainly wouldn't have been able to squat and get up and down off the floor. Because we worked her through these changes, her quality of life has improved in so many ways.

A Better Athlete

You may not identify yourself as an athlete, but you should. You don't have to do sports to be an athlete; it simply means you are using all the basic movements that you are capable of as a human. If you continue to work to be a better athlete, even if you're 60 years old or 60 lbs over weight, you will see progress.

With proper training, you can and should be an athlete. Again, this just means you get good at doing basic movements that translates to better health. If you work with a great tool, like the kettlebell, you'll be doing just that. You'll move better and feel better.

Move Better, Feel Better

Working out has nothing to do with **MOBILITY**, and that's a problem.

You can work out for hours a week and get worse mobility. Ask someone whose only exercise is running to touch their toes– PROBLEM!

Ask a male weight lifter to put his arms over his head– PROBLEM!

And on the opposite end of the spectrum, ask someone who sits at a desk all day and never works out to hold good posture all day and to do a good squat– PROBLEM!

These are all mobility issues, and most Americans have them. The client who has mobility problems is the one that comes into our classes and says, "I can't do kettlebells, they're dangerous for my back."

No, you've gotten so out of shape, your core is so weak because you don't lift heavy things, and your mobility is so bad that doing normal human movements like a kettlebell swing (mimicking picking up something heavy from the ground, or the jumping motion) makes you nervous.

The issue is not the exercise, it's that your body has gotten both WEAK from not exercising for so long, and STIFF from not moving your body the way it's supposed to. Go to a doctor, and they'll often say something like, "Weights aren't right for you. You need some low-impact workouts like water aerobics." Dumb, dumb, dumb.

Look, if this is you, you got here by being too easy on your body. The answer is not to be even easier on it. Doctors say this because they are worried about lawsuits so they're overly conservative, and many of them don't take time to learn about proper exercise programs. The answer is simple. I just said it. Build a base of strength, and get your mobility back.

So now let's explain mobility. If you want some very high-level, scientific explanation of mobility, you're better off with a Physical Therapy text. I'd recommend anything from Gray Cook.

But for the purposes of this book, I'm talking about the ability to move your body the way it's supposed to without pain or restriction. Can you put your arm straight up over your head, elbow locked and bicep next to your ear? Can you squat, butt below your knees, knees in line with your toes and not beyond them? Those are two of the best examples of mobility issues that we see from out of shape people or people who've "worked out" for years.

Training is about MOBILITY. Working out is not. To train means to get better at movements and to move better with less restriction and pain. Your primitive body wants to be trained to use its full range of motion. Your primitive body is built to have great mobility late into life.

Yes, you will possibly lose some mobility or range of motion as you age, but it's a lot less than you think. Just look at elderly people in India. They've gone to the bathroom through a hole in the floor their whole life. At 80, they can still do a better squat than the average 30 year old American. They have great hip mobility because they never stopped using their hips correctly.

The issue here is this. If you don't keep good mobility, then your body will tell you not to move the way it's designed. Let's say your shoulder won't let you press overhead (usually an issue with your upper back– thoracic spine– not your actual shoulder).

That same person then tries to put something heavy into a high shelf in their house, or they play tennis with a friend. Bam! They tear their rotator cuff. Is it because they were too old to do these things? Some would probably say so. But that's picking the wrong issue.

The issue is that they lost proper mobility. You should be able to do basic movements without tearing your rotator cuff. But if you don't train your body and keep it mobile, you will get these types of injuries. So you have a choice. Train to be strong and mobile, or sit and lose it. Or sign up for that great low-impact class at the gym and Think that you're doing something "safe" for your age group.

Summary of 39 Minute Primitive Fitness System

1. **Pick up heavy things**—learn a good core of full-body, multi-joint exercises

2. **Lift explosively for a better heart, bones and butt**—but don't skip out on good, fun steady-state workouts too. Walking, running, swimming or playing your favorite sport are all part of proper health.

3. **Pick the right frequency and intensity**—3-5 days a week, but NOT all the same intensity

4. **Train, don't work out**—workout to build better function, muscle tone or fat burn. Do not work out to leave yourself a puddle on the floor. It's not good for you day after day

Couple this with the Nourishment Plan, and you will completely transform your body, health and emotional life in a matter of weeks to months. Now it's time to talk about how to carry through with the plan and reach your goals.

Chapter 8

Use the 39 Minute GPS to Achieve Your Goals

"I'm Going to be Healthy this Year" is Not a G-O-A-L

YOU HEAR THIS EVERY YEAR around the New Year. Hundreds of thousands of well meaning Americans set out to lose weight and "get healthy," whatever that is. But they never make it clear what healthy is, they don't make real goals that are measurable or objective, and they don't script the steps for success.

So here's how it goes:

> » Day 1– Goal: I'm going to get healthy and eat better. Sally goes to the gym all excited.

The crowds are almost unbearable, but she's determined. At lunch, she orders a salad!

» Day 7– She's getting bored, but she's still going strong. She has that goal, and she's not failing this time.

» Day 14– Her eating has slipped. She's eating out again and sneaking in deserts that she said she was giving up. She's made three out of five workouts this week, but hey, that's still pretty good

» Day 24– Her son is home sick from school. She forgot to shop and meal plan this weekend, so it's back to canned and packaged stuff that's easy to make. She hasn't been to the gym in five days because she's getting busy at work and home.

» Day 37– Sally has given in. She's not admitted to herself yet, but her good attempt has run out of steam. She only goes back to the gym sporadically for the rest of the year, and she doesn't lose any more weight.

This is basically the same story for hundreds of thousands of Americans every year, and that makes me sad. The average person who joins a gym goes for somewhere around 5 weeks before they disappear. Gyms know this very well, so they flood the gates in January, collect their membership contracts, and then watch the numbers drop off by February. Thank you, I'll take that check.

That's a big factor that drives me to write this book and develop the **39 Minute Workout** system. I am sick of watching people with serious health goals try and fail, when the answers are so easy. But as I said, the fat loss industry doesn't make it easy. They make it cost effective for themselves.

If you want to stop this cycle and NEVER SIGN A GYM MEMBERSHIP AGAIN, then you've got to learn how to make real goals and carry through with them. Do that, and follow the **39 Minute Treatment, Training, and Nutrition Systems**, and YOU WILL reach your goals.

Before you start our program, you've got to define your goal. There are a few keys to a good goal:

» **It's got to be big enough to motivate you**– If you're not emotionally invested, forget about it

» **Make it specific and objective**– Good goals are measurable or objective. I'll lose 20 lbs by August. I'll drop two dress sizes. I'll complete a 10k by next spring. I'll get into a two-piece at the beach this summer. These may not be emotionally charged enough for you. Make sure you REALLY want this goal

» **Create your Steps**– If you're hoping to reach this goal but you don't define what you'll do to get there, very specifically, forget about it. There have to be specific tasks/steps you'll follow

» **Build in Accountability**– We do a ton of this for our clients. If you're on your own, you've got to get creative here, but there must be accountability. If it's all on you, you're trusting your will power to get through, and that's risky

Let's break these down in order:

1. **Making BIG Goals & Making them Objective**

In our weight loss challenges at **39 Minute Workout**, the very first thing we do together is nail down our goals. I take every client through the process of making their goals objective, big enough to strive for, and reasonable.

I find that most people dream too small, or don't know how to make objective goals. Some easy ones are around specific measurements. Even though I honestly HATE the scale and wish this wasn't the barometer you use, it does make for a very objective tool, and most of my clients care a lot about the number on the scale.

So starting with a measurable goal is a good objective tool. Pick a weight you'll lose, or number of inches or dress sizes you'll lose. Personally, I'd rather you focus on inches, because this is usually a better sign of success.

Here's the issue with your bodyweight as a barometer for success. I'll share a common scenario I've experienced with my clients at our initial consult.

David: "So Jane, what goals do you have?"
Jane: "I want to drop 50lbs."
David: "When were you last 50lbs lighter?"
Jane: "Um, I think right about when I finished college."

Ok, so Jane is now 44, she's had two children, and she would like to get back to her post-college weight. I hate to be a downer, but NOT going to happen. Have you hung out at a college campus recently? 20 Year olds are just smaller (at least the ones who aren't obese yet).

Even if you've stayed in great shape for 24 years, very few people will be the same weight even 10 years later, especially after having kids. Your body just changes. Look, I wrestled 142 lbs. in High School. I weigh 205 now! There's no way I'm getting back to 142. Even after the Appalachian Trail I was still 165, and I was SKINNY.

So if you're going to make body weight the marker, be reasonable. A good trainer has looked at hundreds of people. I can help you determine a reasonable marker and amount of time to get there.

And as I said before, I would rather you use inches lost or dress sizes dropped as a marker. If you follow my plan, you will put on a little lean muscle, drop a bunch of body fat, and be firm all over. You will absolutely see amazing changes in how your body looks and feels and what size clothes you're wearing.

Let me make it clear. If you have dropped inches and not a bunch of pounds, you've absolutely burned body fat off. And you've replaced it with firmer, healthier lean muscle that keeps you burning more calories and staying lean. As long as you stay active with your **39 Minute Fitness System**, you will hold these positive physical changes as long as you like.

It might sound a bit contradictory, but I also want your goal to be BIG! If your goal isn't big, and particularly if it doesn't carry enough emotion, you won't push hard.

In a phenomenal book on making change, <u>Switch: How to Change Things When Change Is Hard</u>, written by Chip and Dan Heath, they describe your mind as having two aspects. You are an Elephant and a Rider.

The Elephant is your emotional mind, and it's got a distinct strength and weakness. It runs by emotion, so it needs to be excited and motivated, but it also gets easily discouraged.

The Heath brothers explain that when you're making a goal, you've got to make it BIG enough to motivate the Elephant. Here's what this means: If I ask your goal and you say some stock answer that isn't really exciting, you're far less likely to put in the effort it will take to get there.

Your goal needs to be something that REALLY matters to you. I'll give an example. I asked a client in our meeting what her goal is. She says to drop 35 lbs. OK, that might be reasonable, but is it exciting? I ask into more. Why is that important to you? What would it mean to be 35 lbs less? She tells me that she loves to wear summer dresses but she's been embarrassed to do so since she's gained weight. She hates when people walk behind her because she's embarrassed with how she looks.

BAM! That's the emotion. She might get bored with losing 35lbs, but get her picturing what life would be like if she was taking a stroll on the boardwalk with her husband, wearing that cute summer dress and feeling 100% confident... THAT has Emotion.

So this became the heart of her goal. We kept the pounds lost as part of the goal, because that's objective and we'll know when she gets there, but we've also included feeling confident in her summer dress. I like a mixture of objective and subjective, as long as the subjective ones have emotion.

2. **Create Your Steps to Success:**

So you've got a goal that's objective and emotional. Now it's time to create the steps to get you there. For any goal worth striving for, you've got to make some sacrifice and effort.

Back to the Elephant and the Rider, the Rider is our logical brain. It needs order, lists and steps to follow. If you don't "direct the Rider" as the Heath brothers suggest, you have no idea what tasks to focus on.

Writing steps that are specific is where most people fail. This goes back to the original quotes I used. "I'm going to eat better." That is not a step. There's nothing specific about this whatsoever. Your brain will not be clear on what you're supposed to do. Plus, if you don't have a philosophy around nutrition like I've provided for you, "eating better" may not get you anywhere.

So let's talk about good steps. The key here is to pick only a few steps at a time, make them very clear, and stick to the plan.

DO NOT try to tackle too many changes all at once. It will make success very difficult. This might seem like a good idea, but you'll find it very hard to carry through with all of them week after week. Then when you have setbacks, you'll start to judge yourself, see it as failure, and start backing out.

I want you to pace yourself. I would start with one around exercise, and two around nutrition. Something like:

a) I will attend **39 Minute Workout** sessions three times a week

b) I will eat three meals and at least one snack every day

c) I will fill out my food journal every day at the breakfast table after I'm done eating

You see I've chosen one around exercise frequency, one around a specific nutrition step (and one of the most important in my mind), and one that will enable you to keep accountable in the food journal?

Even if you don't have someone to check your food journal, although you should, the act of keeping one is priceless. There's so much research on food journals showing that when people are keeping them, they are much more responsible with their eating. One explanation is that once you see what you are eating every day, it's hard to wonder why you've gained weight. The simple act of seeing everything you eat on paper will usually start to wake you up to changes that need to happen.

Then down the road when you've been awesome at going to class every week, and you're getting all your meals and snacks, you can add another step or two. Master one, add one. Keep that pace up and you'll see huge change.

***If you hit a crisis week due to family or work stress, setbacks in your weight loss, or any other external factor, keep it simple. If you hit a bad phase, and you will along the way, the worst thing to do is get complicated. Drop back to just one or two things you can control, and do them. When you start to come out of your funk, add some steps back.

Another piece to note is the third step above. In Switch, the Heath brothers describe a tool they call an Action Trigger. I used this tool in the third step around filling out a food journal.

If you've got a specific step that you find difficult to follow through with, particularly filling out food journals or going to class, use the tool of the Action Trigger to give your brain clear instructions.

Here are the cliff notes. Instead of saying, "I'll go to **39 Minute Workout** three times a week," tell yourself exactly when you'll go and what will trigger that action.

If you exercise before work, it could be "I'll head to class at 6:15, Monday, Wednesday, and Friday right after I make my smoothie. Then your brain knows, once that smoothie is blended, it's time to head to class.

I'm sure you can make stronger triggers than that example, but USE THIS TOOL. As I said, most Americans start and stop routines within the first month or two, so consistency is an issue for most. You've got to give yourself a good shot at sticking with the plan. So create a laser effective Action Trigger that will tell your brain, "it's time for class."

Examples:

> » Right after I drop my son off at school

> » Once I clock out at work

> » Lay your exercise clothes out in the bathroom. After you shower, seeing them is the trigger to get going

3. **Build a Wall of Accountability Around You**

   As I said, if you can't join our program, you've GOT to figure out how to build accountability into your system. In our system, we've got about 10 layers of accountability built in so that you basically have to fight not to succeed.

If you're doing this on your own, you need to explore some more creative techniques. Here are a few good ones:

» Get a buddy

» Fill out a food and exercise journal

» Reward system

Some of our best success stories have come from people who "buddied up" with another person in our **39 Minute Workout** community. If you are alone and can't join us, this is practically a must.

Look for a buddy who also has a big goal, who you work well with, and who you feel will push you hard and not except excuses. Do not find someone that will be a yes-man or a pushover, because they will do you no good.

Once you've got a buddy, make sure you both have very clear goals and steps defined to reach those goals. Then choose how often you will check in on each other, workout, or meal plan and shop for food. Make any part of this system part of your work together.

Like I said, meal plan together. This is a great way to have success, and this is also one of the pieces my clients struggle with. People really struggle finding time to create good meals, and having a buddy to knock them out with will help you stay fresh and motivated.

You should expect to talk with your buddy at

least twice a week, if not more. Make sure you're asking about the steps they're following, what they're slacking on, and push them. Make an agreement from the start that you will both hold each other to your goals. Then use a mixture of tough love and empathy. **But stay light on the empathy, or it will turn into excuses.**

You don't have to know everything about weight loss to be a good buddy. You've got this book, and you know what to do. Having a decent plan and sticking with it is 100% better than having a perfect plan that you don't follow. So get a buddy and get working.

As I said, a food journal is another form of accountability. Even if you're alone, you will build in personal accountability when you stick with this. You've got my system to follow, and you can grade your own journal. Stick with this for at least 6 weeks, and you'll have built a great base for good habits.

If you've got weight to lose, when you see 2 lbs coming off every week, that's when you know you're on track. If you're below this, nutrition is key. Stick with the food journal and be 100% honest. Pounds WILL come off when you are eating with the plan, I promise.

Some of our clients have successfully used a reward system to motivate themselves to lose a chunk of weight too. I've seen two specific rewards work, but I'd be careful with the second.

The first one is buying clothing that you can't fit in yet or don't feel comfortable wearing– like a great pair of jeans, a new dress, or a bathing suit you're not ready to flaunt– then working toward fitting in it as soon as possible.

This is great Elephant motivation. Remember, the Elephant loves momentum, and strong desire will help feed it. So pick a piece of clothing and motivate yourself with the reward of looking great in it.

The second one is allowing yourself a certain food or drink when you lose a specific amount of weight. For example, if you love beer, you may need to stop drinking it altogether while you're in fat loss mode. But I don't encourage people to give up their favorite food or drink for life. So you could say, "I won't drink a single beer until I lose 20 lbs. And at that point, I'll allow myself two beers, two nights a week."

You see that in this scenario, you've given yourself a very specific reward, a target to shoot for that's motivating, and a specific number of days and drinks you CAN have once you reach that goal. It's important to note that even though I've said that you can go back to drinking, you're not saying "I'll drink as much as I want any day of the week." If you want to lose weight and keep it off, you'll need to exercise limitations around food and drink for the rest of your life.

Conclusion:

If you jump the gun and get into a routine today without doing these first three steps, you're robbing yourself of future success. STOP NOW and write out some good objective goals, a few precise steps, and how you'll build accountability into your routine.

> » **Write a few Goals** that are 1) Objective and/ or 2) Have strong emotion for you. One goal may be objective, and another may have strong emotion

> » **Create Three Steps** you'll follow every day for the first month

> » **Build a wall of Accountability**—Food log, buddy, and/or reward

PILLAR THREE

TREATMENT

CHAPTER #9

WHY ALTERNATIVE THERAPY SHOULD BE YOUR PRIMARY CARE IF YOU LIVE IN THE WESTERN HEMISPHERE

Consistent Acupuncture Treatment is KEY to long-term health, happiness, and symptom free living.

TREATMENT? WHAT'S TREATMENT, AND WHAT in the world does this have to do with weight loss and health?

There's still a strong bias in our culture against traditional medicine. As an acupuncturist, I can't tell you how many times I've gotten the question, "Does acupuncture really work?" That's about as fun of a question as when my 8 month pregnant wife is asked if she's having twins!

Um, yes acupuncture does work. It's "worked" for the last 3,000 years, and it's still the primary care of choice for a huge portion of people on the planet today.

My family uses the three pillars of health as their primary care medicine, and I think you should too. Acupuncture and massage are two of the tools that we use to treat ourselves. We are able to have very inexpensive healthcare and only use doctors when bigger issues arise. I teach all my clients how to do the same, and those that embrace this shift in mentality find a major change in how they view their health.

Modern medicine, also called allopathic medicine, looks at the body in a very strange way. Here are a few places where their perspective is strange, and I believe, has negatively impacted the way Americans view their own health.

>> I've got Type 2 diabetes– let's find a cure

>> I'm 100lbs overweight– let's staple your stomach… or you've got a thyroid problem, let's medicate

>> I'm depressed– let's take meds that make everything gray and blah

>> I've got the sniffles– let's take a medicine cabinet full of drugs to knock it down

And in all these scenarios, there is no talk of the OBVIOUS solution. Here's how alternative medicine would look at these same four symptoms:

» Type-2 diabetes– You're eating and lifestyle are causing disease. Let's fix how you nourish yourself and start losing body fat

» 100lbs overweight– Again, eating and lifestyle are causing significant health problems. Let's put you in control

» Depression– Let's strengthen your body and mind so that you can face this disease. Let's find what days you're stronger, what activities and lifestyles lead to betterment and worsening of your symptoms. If you still need the support of medications, let's work with a progressive doctor to keep you at the minimum dose

» I've got the sniffles– Make your immune system stronger through nourishment, alternative therapy, and herbs

What's the major difference between the first and second scenario? In the first, YOU ARE NOT RESPONSIBLE! You have a symptom, let's "cut it out or medicate it so it goes away."

In the second, you are in control and you have choice. Yes, stuff happens, but you have power and you can take better care of your health.

And here's another obvious problem besides the mentality around health issues I described above. Just like in the fat loss industry that I *EXPOSED* in chapter 1, there's another set of behemoth industries at the heart of our health and medical epidemic: The pharmaceutical and health insurance industries.

Let me tell you a BIG secret. You can make a lot more money from constantly finding very expensive new tests, medications, and surgeries than from telling someone to drink more water, work out and eat grass-fed beef.

Before I ostracize every medical professional on the face of the planet, which I don't mean to do...there's a very big difference between the big industries and their motivations, and the value of modern medicine. There is absolutely a time and place for modern surgeries, medications and tests. There is a place for them, and God forbid I ever get cancer, I will want them.

My issue is with the philosophy that has taken power out of the consumer's hand, and I believe many doctors and nurses are concerned with this trend too. That's why many doctors are opting out of the health insurance, medication pushing nightmare for direct pay options with the consumer. I believe many doctors and nurses are just as disgusted as I am with the trends in healthcare.

The Consumer is SCREAMING for Options

Even in the face of multibillion dollar pharmaceutical and health insurance industries, the consumer is screaming for options. Under the smug and oblivious watch of the modern medical industry who assumed they had the corner market on health, traditional medicine has snuck in and taken the eye of the consumer.

Traditional Medicine (all primitive forms of medicine including acupuncture, herbs, Ayurveda, massage, etc.) have grown to be a multi-billion dollar industry thanks to the consumer. Paying out of pocket for a myriad of options, you the consumer are demanding better options for your health.

I meet so many people at **39 Minute Workout** who want real options for their health, and they do not want another "quick fix" surgery or medication.

I don't think they know it, but what they really want is CONTROL. They want to be told they have the power to change, they are responsible for their health and nobody but them can change.

You absolutely have the power to take control of your health. All you need are the right tools. In this whole book, I've shown you all the garbage the food, weight loss, and medical industry have sold you, and it has all done damage to you and your health. But I believe that if you're still reading, you're looking for a strong path to better health.

What's a Needle got to do with Weight Loss?

I'll bet you'd like me to tell you that I've got an acupuncture point that will make you lose weight! Sorry to burst your bubble, but I'd be a millionaire if I'd found that, and I would be on The Oprah Winfrey Show if it still existed, and I'd be the new Dr. Oz...

Sorry, but it doesn't work that way. But here's what I can help you with.

Weight gain is a function of several factors:

» Type and quantity of food you consume

» Quality of exercise you get

» Stress level/ Emotional health

» Function of your inner organs

I cannot help you much with the first two with treatment, but I can do major changes for the last two. And the cool thing is when we get the third and fourth one under control, this will make major changes in your cravings… so I actually can help the first bullet too!

Your Mind and Nervous system AREN'T built for Today's Pace

You are not built to endure the pace of society. Remember, you are still in the same primitive body and mind that they wore 100,000 years ago. I don't care how cool or helpful modern technology is, or how FUN our world is today, you are not built for this pace.

We always assume that our primitive ancestors worked all day to survive, that their life was a constant struggle, and that they didn't live very long because of this. Wrong, wrong and wrong.

Of course some of this depends on which group of people you're talking about, but for the most part, the rough and tumble life we picture is a bit of a country western tale.

In the book, Limited Wants, Unlimited Means, the author, John Gowdy, describes how much "work" primitive people actually did— The conclusion? A whopping 2-3 hours a day! How about that? I would take that life. Yes, they worked for a few hours a day, leaving the rest of the time to be with family and community, spend time developing art, culture, and spiritual traditions. Not quite the stressful, dangerous life we read about in books.

Let's compare that with your life. You probably sleep less than 8 hours, many of you laughing at that number now... maybe more like 5 or 6...You wake up, make lunches for your kids, rush around for two hours taking care of them, endure the stressful roads, then off to work for 9 hours minimum with stressful deadlines and human interaction, get home, make dinner, get the kids homework done, then get MAYBE two hours to sit down and enjoy life.

Let me state this again. You are not built for this type of stress. Your body and mind do not know how to handle this pace, burdensome and relentless responsibility, lack of creative and quality time with family and friends, and lack of real nourishment and exercise. Your body isn't equipped to multitask and thrive under stress for long periods of time. So if you're used to living with high stress, you're making it that much harder to lose weight.

What ensues after years of living like this depends on who you are and how you cope. Many end up with symptoms of emotional and physical stress, like depression, fatigue, digestive disorders, etc. So you rush to the doctor to "fix" it. Put tape over the warning light on your dashboard, and keep pushing.

How to Squash Your Weight Loss Goals

If your goal is weight loss, a stressful lifestyle will make it very hard to find success. Hormone balance is beyond the scope of what I'm teaching in this book, but you will find clues to stress and squashed weight loss if you look up adrenal exhaustion. It is my belief that stress is the "hidden" cause that hinders weight loss in many people today.

Without going into the science behind adrenal fatigue, suffice it to say that a life of high stress, poor nutrition, poor exercise and poor sleep will make it very hard to drop weight. Your body simply goes into its primitive response to stress, which as I've said before, is to shut down weight loss. It's perceived as a time of struggle, so the body wants to store up. Notice in medical discussion of adrenal exhaustion, the typical body-type is a layer of fat around your middle. Very interesting!

Riding this Roller Coaster Won't Get You there Either

The emotional roller coaster is just as damaging as a stressful lifestyle. In your body, it's all seen as stress, and I can't tell you how many people are emotionally stressed these days. If this is you, you are not alone in the least.

If you struggle with emotional balance, whether you're diagnosed with a disease like depression or bi-polar disorder, or you just suffer with challenging mood and emotional swings, your body is living under constant stress.

Let's look at Melissa's story to show you how emotional challenges effect weight loss and health. Melissa came to us one year ago, and like most of our clients, she had a good bit of weight to lose. But even more apparent, she was sad and not terribly emotionally resilient. It seemed that every little thing that happened to her hit her heart directly.

Melissa started with our kettlebell classes, but the real change came when she started acupuncture treatment with me. In the first few sessions, she couldn't go two minutes without ending up in tears. She slowly grew to trust me, and she shared her pain and challenges. It was apparent that we had a lot of work to do to get her feeling stable and strong.

Melissa, like all my other clients, had all the potential in the world to lose weight. Nothing was stopping her but herself. She was overeating, eating the wrong stuff, and taking everything to heart in her personal life. This affected her feeling of security, her ability to date, and her confidence at work.

But for some reason, she would not follow through with any lasting changes in her nutrition. She knew exactly what she needed to do, but as she would tell you today that she was being stubborn. She also believed she "deserved" to lose weight because she was now working out and drinking more water. And I'll tell you that your body doesn't care what you deserve, it cares what you put into it.

Slowly, over a few months, I started to see Melissa's real character. She was happy and funny. She had a zany sense of humor, and loves to blurt out random thoughts...which get her into trouble sometimes...but it's hilarious.

I could really see her spirit shine by the fall of 2011, but she was still not making the choices she needed to with eating. BUT, her life was improving. She wasn't crying anymore in treatment, she wasn't emotionally raw and vulnerable, and when there were stressful changes at work, her response was so different now. This confident and strong woman was coming out.

And all good stories have a happy ending. As I write this book, we're coming to the end of our third body weight challenge of the year, and Melissa is going to WIN! I won't say it was easy, but she finally started to do what she was capable of doing all along. Now, week after week she's dropping about 2 lbs, and her body is shrinking before our eyes. She finally knows she can do it.

When you ask her what she attributes her change too, it was the support of her **39 Minute Workout** community, it was the workout and nutrition, but for her, it was the acupuncture that made the biggest change in her life and emotional health. I'm so proud of her, and I look forward to her continued progress.

What PATTERN do You Suffer From?

In acupuncture, we treat what we call "patterns." In the bullet list above, I talked about four factors of weight loss, and the last one is the function of your internal organs. I'm sure if you're only use to western medicine that sounds bizarre. But when I explain some of the patterns acupuncture can help you with, it will make more sense.

Patterns all have one thing in common, and we all have one or more of them challenging our health. Just like the concept of homeostasis, our body is in a constant battle to remain stable. How we treat ourselves through lifestyle makes the biggest impact on this, but sometimes, there are things beyond our control.

For one, we don't all choose the stress we live with. It's easy to say "you need to work less and sleep more." But if you're a single mom and you've got to have two jobs to keep afloat, that's not a reality.

There are other factors, such as environmental degradation affecting our food, water and air that we are exposed to, and we can't completely avoid this. And some people, even if they take wonderful care of their health, will struggle with emotional challenges. Stuff happens. We might lose our job, lose a loved one, or develop a disease. We don't have control of everything that happens.

All of these factors impact our health and our ability to lose weight. So let's discuss a few of the most common ones that you might suffer with.

Dampness/ Weak Spleen

For women, I'd say this is the most common and concerning pattern making weight loss challenging. The primary cause of dampness is simple; overconsumption of damp foods! I've described dampness earlier, but here's the list again:

» Dairy

» Sugar

» Wheat

» Cold and too much raw food

Basically, damp foods are everything I've told you not to eat. They're also the center of the American diet, especially for children. If you think about the word dampness, you can imagine the symptoms.

» Feeling of lethargy— particularly after meals

» Heavy limbs

» Bloated stomach and slow digestion

» Cloudy/slow thinking

» Squishy flesh

This is a huge challenge, because the center of our diet is damp foods. That's why it's so important you learn the Primitive Nourishment philosophy. If you don't work to get dampness in check, it will make weight loss very challenging.

If you clean out damp foods for just 5 days, take note of what your flesh feels like. For most people, you'll see a positive change in how firm your skin and flesh are in just a few days.

But long-term dampness can be very challenging to clear with diet alone. If you've eaten like this for years and have any of the symptoms in the above list, you'll find it a lot slower to heal. Acupuncture will speed that process up dramatically.

With acupuncture, we can encourage the body to clear the dampness held in your body. You'll see positive changes in digestion, bloating, allergies (often associated with dampness), and your clarity of thought.

Over the long-term, with consistent treatment, we can help your body's Spleen function improve too. A weak Spleen (that's the Chinese medical concept of Spleen I described before when discussing digestion of processed foods) is to blame for challenges in weight loss and food transformation. Basically, if you've got a weak Spleen you'll lack the physical strength you're capable of having, lack digestive strength making it tougher to turn food into energy, and this will lead to a much harder time dropping weight.

With acupuncture, we can strengthen your Spleen and reduce dampness together, which will unlock your potential to get more out of your fitness and nourishment efforts. If you're just working the first two pillars, you can still lack the internal organ strength and health to make great use of those changes. Use consistent treatment to TURN UP the power of your fat burn!

Kidney Yin Deficiency

Basically everyone in our culture has some level of Kidney yin deficiency. We're overworked and under rested, but we also lack the proper nourishment to deal with this constant onslaught of stress. So our Kidneys, sort of like our central battery of energy, get worn down.

The symptoms of Kidney yin deficiency are:

» Frequent feeling of tiredness

- » Night sweats, hot flashes
- » Dizziness or tinnitus
- » Poor memory
- » Weak/sore back
- » Achy bones
- » Constipation

The person who suffers most with this pattern feels chronically tired, and tends towards back aches and weakness. They are often people who Go-Go-Go! But the flip side is that they have nothing left in the tank. So they're either going, or they're collapsing.

This person will find it VERY hard to lose weight unless she creates balance. If she doesn't use her reserves wisely, and if she doesn't take time to regenerate her energy she will just wear down. Weight loss becomes virtually impossible until this pattern is put in check.

This is the pattern that best fits me, so I can see it very clearly in someone else. And what's the toughest thing about helping this type of person??? They are addicted to always pushing hard in their life. Telling them to slow down is like telling them to die. They don't want to, and they aren't very easy to convince otherwise.

Acupuncture really is the best tool to help this pattern. You can tell someone until you're blue in the face to slow down and rest more, but that usually falls on deaf ears. Treatment with a 5-element acupuncturist (my form of training) will help this person create boundary around her use of energy reserves.

Treatment has an amazing way of bringing balance to people. It helps them see and feel more clearly how their lifestyle is affecting their health and quality of life, and most people begin making better decisions because of it. It's amazing how reasoning with people with this pattern is as good as pounding your head against the wall, but treatment can get them to actually slow down and make better use of their energy.

As I said before, we aren't built to deal with the stress of modern culture. The person with Kidney yin deficiency will particularly suffer from the pace and excessive responsibility that life requires of us today. And this will make it hard for them to lose weight. This pattern goes hand-in-hand with the western diagnosis of adrenal exhaustion, and both make weight loss challenging. So if this is you, go find a practitioner who can help you get it under control.

Stagnant Liver Qi

There are two words that come to mind with the person who suffers from stagnant Liver Qi (pronounced Chee). Frustrated and tight!

Here's a quick list of symptoms associated with it:

- » Feeling of distention/tightness in belly or diaphragm area

- » Depression and moodiness— quick to anger

- » Nausea, poor appetite, belching

- » Irregular and painful periods

As you see, there's tightness in the belly and muscles, and a level of frustration which leads to moodiness— usually depression or fits of anger. This person is bound up and needs to exercise VERY badly. Movement is an absolute requirement for her, because she's got to smooth out and burn off some of that tight, hot energy.

Someone with this symptom needs to be very careful with alcohol consumption, and other foods that make them hot or more frustrated. Alcohol is the Achilles heel for them, as it breeds more stagnation, anger, pain or tightness.

The words for them should be SMOOTH and CALM. And while exercise will play a big role in creating this, treatment will play an integral role too. Acupuncture is the single most powerful tool at smoothing out the frustration and tightness of stagnant Liver qi. Again, we can speed up the process of healing a lot faster than you can with nutrition and movement alone.

If this person has a challenge losing weight, it's most likely to do with poor digestion and stress levels. Because they tend to bloat, they are prone to storing extra fluid and distention in their bellies. Then as it usually goes, they'll crave all the wrong foods and drinks to "treat" the symptoms.

Making good food choices can be very challenging for them. We tend to crave what we least need. The person with dampness probably LOVES cheese/dairy. The person with Kidney yin deficiency probably LOVES coffee. And the person with stagnant Liver qi probably loves alcohol.

We can Treat these Patterns Together

The acupuncturist can help get these patterns in control so that you STOP craving and doing what is least productive for your health. Wording that in the positive, we can help you feel more in tune with your body so that you find it easier to make good lifestyle decisions.

All of these patterns can be handled and treated. Each one can be treated by an acupuncturist, and your practitioner can help you find the best foods and lifestyles to support your healing. But skipping out on the third pillar of health will greatly hinder your speed of recovery and overall health.

Whether your goal is weight loss or simply living the healthiest life you can, acupuncture will support you. As I've said before, in a world of ultra-expensive and invasive medications and surgeries, most of what you suffer from should be dealt with by the Three Pillars of Health.

"Primary care" as we call it should really be acute care for severe symptoms like broken bones and cancer. In the realm of your daily health over a lifetime, alternative medicine has far better answers and solutions for you.

THE MENTAL TRANSFORMATION

What do YOU Truly Value

Y OU'LL PAY FOR WHAT YOU value. So where do you spend your money? What's the PRICE you're willing to pay for health?

I meet people every week who want so badly to be healthy, to lose the weight they've carried for years, and to be happy and content in their lives. But then it comes…the price conversation.

I've found there are two distinct groups of people; those that would buy a nice car any day of the week, but then balk at the price of taking care of their health. Then there are the folks like my clients who value health as a top priority.

The latter group values health and quality of life, so that's where they spend their money. They would never balk at making an investment in their health, because nothing matters if you're not well.

Spending on health doesn't always seem "sexy." It's fun to buy a new car or go on a vacation, but having great health or buying 10 acupuncture sessions may not feel as fun. You can't drive it around and show it off. You can't look at it in the driveway and admire it.

But you will get what you value. And if you truly value your health, you'll put your money there. I hear a lot of people say, "Oh, I can't do acupuncture, I already pay for healthcare."

Or my favorite one, "I have 50 lbs to lose, I've carried this weight for 10 years, and I can't lose it on my own, and I'm so tired of living like this." Ok, Jenn, here's my system, here's exactly what we'll do for you and how long it will take for you to get there. We do X, Y, and Z to ensure your good success, and you will achieve this change and hold onto your results unlike the times you've yo-yo'd in the last 10 years. Here's the best package for you."

Client X, "oh, I won't pay that. I've already got a gym membership."

I Want to go to Hawaii

I've got an analogy for the people that think this way about their health and where they invest their money. Whether you're talking about not doing acupuncture because you already pay for healthcare, or not doing our program because you already pay for a gym membership, the question is, DO YOU HAVE THE RIGHT TOOL?

If you tell me you want to make huge, sweeping changes in your health, but you aren't willing to invest the money, it's like this.

"I would like to go to Hawaii."

"Great, here are the travel plans. Here's the plane you'll be flying on, your hotel, dinner package, and lovely spa treatments."

"Oh, but I already own a car!"

Ummm. Ok, you own a car. I don't think that's going to get you where you want. But if you're happy with that, just keep that car and tell me how it goes. Six or twelve months from now when I see you and you're still the same weight, let's talk about that trip to Hawaii again. It might seem more tempting.

I DO intend to be blunt here. The thing is you get what you pay for. You get out of life what you invest in. People who make investments and save money have reserves for troubled times. They tend to carry less stress, and they have better quality of life because they don't carry the stress of always chasing the next paycheck.

The person who worships their car but won't pay for a system to drop 50lbs and revolutionize their health does not think like this. They're always hoping for sunny weather, when they can walk around with those 50 lbs, hoping for the day when they're inspired to go to the gym and get the weight off. But that day never comes for these folks. It comes for the people that make investments in their health.

This leads me to a concept/analogy that I developed called the **Health Portfolio**

The Health Portfolio

In financial planning you've got a Wealth Portfolio, a diverse set of investments that help you bank greater financial freedom for the future. When a family has been responsible with building their portfolio, there's a certain calm that comes over them. If they've truly put in money and invested over time, even with changes in the economy, there's a level of security.

Your health can be treated the same way. You can "bank" good health by making steady deposits day after day, month after month. And the result is a very strong immune system, greater emotional and physical happiness and freedom, and greater peace of mind when things go wrong.

Who do you think feels emotionally stronger when they get the diagnosis of cancer, someone who works out three times a week and eats a Primitive diet for years, or someone who worships the TV, hasn't worked out or taken a walk in years, and lives on pizza and diet Coke?

Nobody wants to get a diagnosis like this, but the reality is, shit happens. And the person who has done more to take care of her health and become in-tune with her body and health over the long haul will have more reserves of emotional and physical strength to deal with crisis.

Of course there are also other applications to the Health Portfolio, too.

I don't think it's any secret that people who take care of themselves have a better quality of life. I'll give you a scenario to consider, and most of my clients have experienced this. You start eating really clean, get on the **39 Minute Workout**, and you're dropping pounds. Months have passed, and for the most part, you are feeling better physically and emotionally than you have in years.

Then you hit the holiday, or a few weeks where you just get away from your eating plan, and you go back to eating like the average American– cereal and milk with coffee for breakfast, fast food for lunch, pizza and soda for dinner.

Within two weeks, you and the people around you start to see changes. You're in a bad mood, you're reactive to the small stuff in life that wasn't bothering you, and you feel bloated and slow.

This is the exact story that one of our clients, we'll call Kathy, experienced this past winter. Kathy has now lost 62 lbs in our system, and she's been through two of our weight loss challenges. But at the end of last fall, for reasons that don't matter here, she went back to the eating that had her significantly overweight and "a walking stroke waiting to happen," as she described herself.

In using our system, Kathy had dropped about 50 lbs by last fall, but in a month of getting away from the program, she got back to her old habits. A few weeks into eating her old way, she reported feeling symptoms of depression, and just feeling junky, bloated and slow inside.

But because Kathy remained tapped into our system, she kept working out, and she got herself right back on the program. Two months later, she's down another 12 lbs or so, and her health is better than it was in her 20's. Those are her words not mine.

This is the value of making constant deposits into your **Health Portfolio**. If you build this portfolio consistently, several things will happen.

1. You'll know when you've gotten away from what was working

2. You're body will tell you it's not happy

3. You'll have the drive and know-how to get your health back

4. Your health will bounce back VERY quickly

If you have not yet started building your portfolio, you'll have to work a lot harder. A year ago, Kathy had to put a ton of hard work in. She had to learn a way of eating that was completely different than before. She had to train in our **39 Minute Workout**, even though her body griped at the hard work with all the weight she was carrying. It was not easy, and many like her came and went, because they just didn't want to put in the effort that Kathy was willing to make.

Kathy is a shining example of someone who changed her priorities and took the bull by the horns. She went from an overweight, unhealthy ticking time bomb, to someone that's built an amazing **Health Portfolio**. She should be applauded for her efforts.

THE WEIGHT LOSS INDUSTRY WANTS YOU FAT... BUT I WANT YOU TO BE FIT

T HE WHOLE PREMISE OF THIS book was to **EXPOSE** the weight loss industry and prove that their intentions are not clean. They do not want you to be leaner or healthier, or there would be better, more simple products that were rooted in nature, time honored truths, and effective.

To the contrary, what they've provided us, the American public, for the last few decades is disgusting, FAST and unnatural foods that are making us sick and obese, weight loss supplements and surgeries, and a thousand workouts and exercise tools that don't deliver.

BUT I want you FIT!

Why does it matter so much to me? First off, I care about the health of you and everyone you know. I care that you have access to information around treatment, training and nutrition that is frankly your birth right. I care that your children grow up in a world where people have gone back to the simple truths of health and fitness that had us lean and healthy for thousands of years.

I don't think that it's acceptable that we should live this way. You should not have to struggle to be lean and healthy. You should not be pitched a thousand useless exercise tools and foods that don't nourish. But frankly, I don't think we're getting anywhere politically and in business. I don't think we can make the change at those levels quickly enough to help you NOW.

Like I said, these tools I've shared are a birth right. You should have access to simple truths around exercise, nutrition and traditional medicine. These tools literally have the ability to transform your physical and emotional health.

I also wrote this book because I feel that people are suffering emotionally. I'm not implying that we all have mental illness, but far too many people suffer from emotional pain on a day-to-day basis— exhaustion, mood swings, sadness in work and family, and frustration. This leads us to live lives that aren't as productive and fulfilling as they can be.

I've seen NOTHING make faster and more effective changes to the quality of one's life than changes in nutrition, exercise, and acupuncture treatment.

I've watched hundreds of clients enter our program

with depression, sadness, anger, sleep issues, incredible weakness in their body, poor sleep, relationship issues, and confidence issues.

If they took the standard approach, they'd try to FIX their issues with drugs and surgery, or they'd just flat out suffer through it. But there is a simple truth— when you eat what nourishes you correctly, get frequent exercise, and fill in the holes in your health with acupuncture, amazing changes are possible very quickly.

I will venture to say that most of what you suffer from emotionally and physically can be cleaned up and improved rapidly with the three pillars. And I say that with over 7 years of experience in helping people make this transformation.

Making Personal
Transformation Easy

My mission is Making Personal Transformation EASY.

As I told you in Chapter 8, a real goal should be big and scary. And this mission is my big goal. It is no small feat to take an American public who have been sold such a load of garbage when it comes to diet, exercise and medicine and help them transform quickly and easily.

I am so passionate about this subject, and I care so much that you can achieve your own health transformation easily because I believe you deserve access to your best health and quality of life possible. I believe you have the right to control your health and happiness, and you've been kept from this full potential by what you've been taught. That part is not your fault.

But that is the mission we live every day at **39 Minute Workout**. Every day my staff and I strive to make transformation easy for our clients. We do this by stripping down all the dogma and barriers in the way. We find what's most important for your health and fitness, find the quickest way there, and guide the process every step of the way.

If I've done my job, this book has acted to do the same. If you've thoroughly read this book and absorbed it, you will now see how easy it is to achieve real physical and emotional balance, and yes, rapid fat loss too.

You do this by following the Three Pillars:

1. **<u>Treatment</u>—Get your "patterns" in check and live at your optimal health. Create greater balance in your organ systems and emotional life**

2. **<u>Training</u>—Find the right balance of intense exercise with weights and calm exercise to burn stress**

3. **<u>Nutrition</u>—Follow the 4 Simple Rules— Frequent, with the season, easily digestible (not processed), and frequent protein**

THE NEW CONVERSATION

I WILL ALSO BE HAPPY IF I've helped change the conversation away from POUNDS and towards HEALTH.

Nourishment instead of Diet.

I do care that you burn all the body fat off your body that you need to be healthy. But here's a little secret. <u>I could care less what you weigh</u>. I know many of you will still care a lot about your weight, and I hope to change that.

Body weight is about as useful to you as calories. STOP caring about it. It means absolutely nothing to your health and even how attractive you look, and I know that's the real motivation for people who care about body weight.

They have a concept in their mind that says, "I've got to weigh X or I won't look/feel attractive." Let me tell you something. If you get firm all over, have nice lean muscle that holds your flesh in, have a kettlebell butt, great skin from being properly nourished, sleep better, etc. you WILL be extremely attractive.

You will have a physical and psychological confidence that will exude from your body and eyes. And nobody will have a freaking clue what you weigh. If you follow the plan, you'll also have the least amount of body fat possible, and you really shouldn't care about anything more than having low body fat (appropriate to YOU), a nice firm body, and the best health you're capable of.

My Expanding Community

I T'S BEEN A COMPLETE JOY to help people in Howard County, Maryland and surrounding communities. I've been privileged to work with hundreds of great people for the last 7 years. I've had the pleasure of watching people live better quality lives, get free of physical and emotional pain, transform their bodies, and get their confidence back.

I've been challenged to learn and stretch myself, to become a student of health and fitness, and to be as useful as possible to as many people as possible.

And now, 7 years in, I've created this system that makes the tools I've discovered even more accessible. With this book I can reach so many more people and spread the word about Primitive Health and Fitness to a much wider community.

Please help me spread this word so that others can find their own, SIMPLE path to health and fitness. Please help me start the Primitive Health and Fitness Revolution! As I showed in Chapter 1, here's the manifesto for change.

The Primitive Health and Fitness Revolution Manifesto:

> » **I will accept personal responsibility**– As a consumer, I accept the fact that I am solely responsible for what I feed myself and my family. While there are many temptations and pitfalls along the way, I am ultimately responsible for my choices.

> » **I will be a wise consumer**– I will demand better products from the farmer to the grocery store. I will know where my food comes from, and I will seek the best possible foods and sources that my budget will allow.

> » **I will educate myself on the Primitive Rules of nutrition and exercise**– I will commit to getting the movement and nutrition that my body needs. I will step out of my comfort zone and explore the exercise that my body needs, even if it seems foreign to me at first.

> » **I will be a role model for my family and others around me**– We cannot make a Primitive Revolution unless we make it viral. We have to spread the word, educate our friends and family, and be a great example.

The fact is, there's an epidemic going on right now. Our culture is sick with obesity, chronic illnesses, and emotional pain, most of which are TREATABLE with the Three Pillars. I am not asking that you pound the pavement and march with me, although that could be fun. All I ask is that you commit yourself to living in line with the manifesto, and that you commit to the pillars.

What's at stake is your family's and your own health and happiness.

I really want to hear from you and to help you make these changes. Please feel free to email me at david@39minuteworkout.com. I want to hear success stories, questions, and words of inspiration.

Dedicated to your health,

David Beares

ABOUT THE AUTHOR

DAVID BEARES holds a unique perspective on health and fitness. He draws from his training as a Licensed Acupuncturist, a certified Russian Kettlebell instructor, his experience hiking the entire Appalachian Trail, and his training in primitive survival skills. This all comes together in a system that he calls the 39 Minute Workout, "Primitive Health and Fitness."